Specialist Training in
ENDOCRINOLOGY

Commissioning Editor: Timothy Horne
Development Editor: Clive Hewat
Project Manager: Jess Thompson
Designer: George Ajayi
Illustration Manager: Bruce Hogarth
Illustrator: Ian Ramsden

Specialist Training in
ENDOCRINOLOGY

EDITED BY

Maurice F. Scanlon BSc MD FRCP

Professor of Endocrinology
Director of the Centre for Endocrine and Diabetes Sciences
School of Medicine
Cardiff University
Cardiff, UK

Aled Rees PhD MRCP

Senior Lecturer
Centre for Endocrine and Diabetes Sciences
School of Medicine
Cardiff University
Cardiff, UK

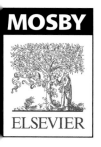

MOSBY

ELSEVIER

Edinburgh   London   New York   Oxford   Philadelphia   St Louis   Sydney   Toronto   2008

MOSBY
ELSEVIER

An imprint of Elsevier Limited

First published 2008

ISBN 978-0-7234-3408-5

British Library Cataloguing in Publication Data
A catalogue record for this book is available from the British Library

Library of Congress Cataloging in Publication Data
A catalog record for this book is available from the Library of Congress

Notice
Knowledge and best practice in this field are constantly changing. As new research and experience broaden our knowledge, changes in practice, treatment and drug therapy may become necessary or appropriate. Readers are advised to check the most current information provided (i) on procedures featured or (ii) by the manufacturer of each product to be administered, to verify the recommended dose or formula, the method and duration of administration, and contraindications. It is the responsibility of the practitioner, relying on their own experience and knowledge of the patient, to make diagnoses, to determine dosages and the best treatment for each individual patient, and to take all appropriate safety precautions. To the fullest extent of the law, neither the Publisher nor the Editors assumes any liability for any injury and/or damage to persons or property arising out or related to any use of the material contained in this book.
The Publisher

    your source for books, journals and multimedia in the health sciences

www.elsevierhealth.com

The publisher's policy is to use **paper manufactured from sustainable forests**

Printed in China

Contents

Contributors

Nazar N. Amso FRCOG PhD ILTHEM
Senior Lecturer / Honorary Consultant
University Hospital of Wales
Cardiff, UK

Justin H. Davies MD FRCPCH MRCP
Consultant Paediatric Endocrinologist
Child Health Directorate
Southampton University Hospital Trust
Southampton, UK

John W. Gregory MD FRCPCH FRCP
Professor in Paediatric Endocrinology
Department of Child Health
Wales College of Medicine
Cardiff University
Cardiff, UK

John H. Lazarus MA MD FRCP FACE FRCOG
Professor of Clinical Endocrinology
School of Medicine
Cardiff University
Cardiff, UK

Amanda O'Leary MRCOG
Subspeciality trainee in Reproductive
Medicine
University Hospital of Wales
Cardiff, UK

Michael D. Page MD FRCP
Consultant Physician
Royal Glamorgan Hospital
Llantrisant, UK

Julia Platts FRCP
Consultant in Diabetes and Endocrinology
Glan Clwyd Hospital NHS Trust
Bodelwyddan, UK

L. D. Kuvera E. Premawardhana MBBS FRCP
Consultant Physician
Caerphilly Miners' Hospital
Caerphilly
Honorary Consultant Physician
University Hospital of Wales
Cardiff, UK

Aled Rees PhD MRCP
Senior Lecturer
Centre for Endocrine and Diabetes
Sciences
School of Medicine
Cardiff University
Cardiff, UK

Maurice F. Scanlon BSc MD FRCP
Professor of Endocrinology
Director of The Centre for Endocrine and
Diabetes Sciences
School of Medicine
Cardiff University
Cardiff, UK

Jamie Smith MD FRCP
Consultant in Diabetes and Endocrinology
Torbay Hospital
Torquay, UK

Preface

This book is intended for doctors new to the management of endocrine disease, especially trainees making the transition from core general medical training to a specialized training programme in endocrinology and diabetes. It is loosely based on the learning needs outlined in the 2003 Joint Committee on Higher Medical Training Curriculum for Endocrinology and Diabetes. Hence it should serve as a useful guide to the management of common endocrine conditions but is not intended as a comprehensive resource and should not be viewed as a replacement for the larger reference texts in the field. We have tried to make it 'user friendly' with an emphasis throughout on the use of illustrations, tables and flow diagrams. History taking, investigation and treatment form the bulk of the text, although brief details on anatomy and physiology and the management of rarer but important conditions are included. Each chapter concludes with self assessment cases which have been taken from the clinic and are intended to reinforce the learning process. We hope that this book will form the first of several editions and welcome any suggestions for improvements.

Aled Rees
Maurice F. Scanlon
Cardiff 2007

Acknowledgements

We are indebted to several colleagues who contributed chapters including Drs Nazar Amso and Amanda O'Leary from the Department of Obstetrics and Gynaecology at the University Hospital of Wales; Dr Justin Davies from the Department of Child Health at Southampton General Hospital; Professor John Gregory from the Department of Child Health at the University Hospital of Wales; Professor John Lazarus from the Centre for Endocrine and Diabetes Sciences at the University Hospital of Wales; Dr Mike Page from the Department of Endocrinology and Diabetes at the Royal Glamorgan Hospital; Dr Julia Platts from the Department of Endocrinology and Diabetes at Glan Clwyd Hospital; Dr Kuvera Premawardhana from the Department of Endocrinology and Diabetes at Caerphilly Miners' Hospital; and Dr Jamie Smith from the Department of Endocrinology and Diabetes at Torbay General Hospital. We thank the Department of Medical Illustration at the University Hospital of Wales for their work with many of the images and are grateful to Professor Leslie de Groot on behalf of Thyroid Disease Manager (www.thyroidmanager.org) for his permission to use the illustrations on thyroid fine needle aspiration. We are especially grateful to the patients who agreed for their images to be published. Finally, thanks to our wives Leanne and Sue for their support.

Pituitary and hypothalamic disease

1

M. Scanlon

The anterior pituitary (AP) gland develops from an upward evagination of the stomadeal ectoderm (Rathke's pouch). This then makes contact with a downward extension of the ventral forebrain (diencephalon), which forms the posterior pituitary (PP). Early AP development and specific cell type differentiation is controlled by sequential activation and interaction of a range of transcriptional, regulatory genes and mutations in each of these cause some of the varied phenotypes of congenital hypopituitarism. In parallel with organogenesis and cell differentiation, the AP develops its own microvascular circulation (the hypophyseal portal system), via which hypothalamic neuropeptides and dopamine (DA), synthesized in neuronal cell bodies in the hypothalamic nuclei, are transported from the median eminence to control the function of specific AP cell types. In contrast, the PP is a direct neuronal extension from the supraoptic and paraventricular nuclei of the hypothalamus, and its hormones are secreted directly into the systemic circulation. The important anatomical relationships are highlighted in Figure 1.1.

PHYSIOLOGY

Growth hormone

Most circulating growth hormone (GH; 75%) is in the form of a single polypeptide chain (191 amino acids) associated with its binding protein, which is identical to the extracytoplasmic portion of the GH receptor. The dominant hypothalamic control of synthesis and release is stimulatory through the phasic interaction of GH-releasing hormone (GHRH, 40 and 44 amino acid forms – stimulatory) and somatostatin (14 and 28 amino acid forms – inhibitory). This produces a variable pulsatile pattern of secretion and a pronounced circadian rhythm, with maximum GH levels at night in association with slow-wave sleep. Several other peptides have GH secretagogue action, particularly ghrelin (28 amino acids), which is found mainly in the stomach and acts (among other things) to stimulate appetite. In this way, GH secretion is involved in the complex interactions in the control of energy expenditure.

GH stimulates the synthesis and release of hepatic insulin-like growth factor (IGF)-1 (70 amino acids) synthesis and release, which exerts negative feedback control over GH

1

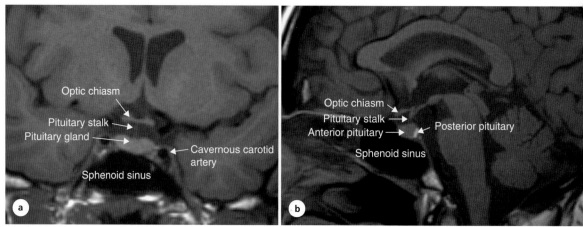

Figure 1.1
Coronal **(a)** and sagittal **(b)** magnetic resonance images of a normal pituitary gland to illustrate the anatomical relationships. Cranial nerves III, IV and VI traverse the cavernous sinus alongside the internal carotid artery. The posterior pituitary shows as a bright signal.

production at hypothalamic–pituitary levels. Only 1% of circulating IGF-1 is free, the rest being associated with a range of binding proteins that play an important role in regulating bioactivity at the tissue level. Overall, GH/IGF-1 secretion gradually declines throughout life, and circulating IGF-1 levels must be interpreted against an age-related reference range. Through the mediation of circulating IGF-1, locally produced IGF-1 and direct local actions, GH exerts a wide range of actions: it is crucial for normal growth and bone development through childhood, adolescence and young adulthood, and it has important stimulatory actions throughout life on protein synthesis, lipolysis, gluconeogenesis and bone metabolism, as well as on drive, energy and general well-being.

Follicle-stimulating hormone and luteinizing hormone

The gonadotrophins form part of a family of dimeric, polypeptide glycoprotein hormones that include thyroid-stimulating hormone (TSH) and chorionic gonadotrophin (placental in origin). Each hormone comprises a common α subunit (94 amino acids) and a hormone-specific β subunit (follicle-stimulating hormone, FSH, 111; luteinizing hormone, LH, 121 amino acids) encoded on different genes. Glycosylation of the intact molecules is essential for full biological activity. The hypothalamus exerts dominant stimulatory control over LH/FSH synthesis and release via gonadotrophin-releasing hormone (GnRH), balanced at hypothalamic–pituitary levels by complex feedback interactions with gonadal steroids (oestradiol, progesterone, testosterone) and a variety of gonadal peptides (inhibin, activin, follistatin).

The regular pulsatile release of GnRH, LH and FSH (every 90 min) is central to normal gonadal function, and anything that disrupts this leads to hypogonadism (e.g. continuous stimulation by GnRH agonists causes desensitization/down-regulation of gonadotrophins and reversible hypogonadism). In women, LH and FSH control cyclical ovulation, with appropriate changes in oestradiol and progesterone secretion. In men, LH stimulates testosterone production by Leydig cells and FSH stimulates spermatogenesis.

Thyroid-stimulating hormone

Like the gonadotrophins, TSH is a dimeric polypeptide glycoprotein hormone comprising both α and β subunits. The dominant hypothalamic control is stimulatory via the tripeptide thyrotrophin-releasing hormone (TRH), balanced by the negative feedback actions of free thyroid hormones at hypothalamic–pituitary levels. Hypothalamic somatostatin, DA and circulating cortisol also contribute to lesser degrees in the inhibitory control of TSH release. TSH secretion displays an ultradian pulsatile pattern with a dominant circadian rhythm, during which circulating levels rise during the evening before the onset of sleep and decline throughout the day (within the reference range). Despite this, thyroid hormone levels remain relatively constant. Normal circulating levels of free thyroid hormones are essential to maintain balanced activity of all cells and tissues.

Adrenocorticotrophic hormone

Adrenocorticotrophic hormone (ACTH) is a 39 amino acid peptide derived from the large precursor peptide pro-opiomelanocortin. Dominant stimulatory hypothalamic control is via corticotrophin-releasing hormone (41 amino acids), balanced by powerful negative feedback inhibition exerted by cortisol at hypothalamic–pituitary levels. Cortisol levels show a transient, minor rise following meals, and there are both ultradian and circadian rhythms in ACTH and cortisol secretion, with levels peaking at around 8 a.m. from a nadir between 8 p.m. and 2 a.m. The hypothalamic–pituitary–adrenal axis plays a central role in maintaining intracellular and metabolic homeostasis in the unstressed state but particularly in response to a wide range of stressors, both physical (e.g. hypoglycaemia; acute, severe disease) and psychological (e.g. depression).

Prolactin

Prolactin (PRL) is a polypeptide hormone with structural similarities to both GH (42% homology) and placental chorionic mammosomatotrophin. In contrast to all other AP hormones, the dominant hypothalamic control of PRL synthesis and release is inhibitory via the neurotransmitter DA, which inhibits adenylate cyclase activity through DA_2 receptors on lactotrophs. PRL has an autoregulatory system via a short-loop positive feedback action on hypothalamic dopaminergic neurons, causing increased DA synthesis and transport to the AP in the face of rising PRL levels.

As with GH, PRL is released acutely in stressful situations (e.g. hypoglycaemia, grand mal epilepsy and even venepuncture in some individuals), and levels rise markedly throughout pregnancy due to increased stimulation of lactotrophs by rising oestradiol levels. The circadian change in PRL secretion parallels that of TSH closely, with levels rising during the evening before the onset of sleep (usually within the reference range). The major action of PRL is to stimulate milk production by breast tissue. Postpartum, suckling causes acute PRL release against the background of sustained hyperprolactinaemia until weaning occurs. This physiological hyperprolactinaemia prevents the return of menses through both hypothalamic (inhibition of GnRH pulsatility) and ovarian (antagonism of the actions of gonadotrophins) actions.

Arginine vasopressin and oxytocin

Arginine vasopressin (AVP; also known as antidiuretic hormone) and oxytocin are small peptides (nine amino acids) synthesized by neurons originating in the hypothalamic supraoptic and paraventricular nuclei. Some paraventricular nuclei neurons terminate at the median eminence and release AVP into hypophyseal portal blood to interact synergistically with corticotrophin-releasing hormone in the control of corticotrophs. In contrast, the so-called magnocellular neurons of the supraoptic and paraventricular nuclei terminate in the PP, where they release AVP and oxytocin directly into the systemic circulation.

The main action of AVP is to control blood volume by reducing free water clearance by the kidney (by increasing the water permeability of tubular cells in the distal nephron), thus producing concentrated urine. Hence the major regulator of AVP secretion is the plasma osmolality via the hypothalamic thirst centre, but AVP release is also increased by marked hypotension, hypovolaemia and vomiting. Oxytocin stimulates smooth muscle contraction in the pregnant uterus and lactating breast but has no clearly established role in men.

HYPOPITUITARISM

Hypopituitarism is due to congenital or acquired deficiency of one or several pituitary hormones. The overall incidence is variably estimated at 10–40 new cases/million per year, but this may be an underestimate because, as yet, there are no comprehensive data about the incidence of GH deficiency in several different situations, for example head injury. Not surprisingly the presentation can be very varied depending on the precise cause (Box 1.1) and degree of hormone deficiency.

Clinical features

These can be non-specific, such as general malaise, lack of energy, tiredness and weight gain and/or relate to specific hormone deficiencies.

GH deficiency

The GH/IGF-1 axis is usually the first to be affected in progressive pituitary disease. Prior to epiphyseal fusion in childhood, deficiency causes short stature and delayed bone

Box 1.1: Causes of hypopituitarism

Tumours

- Pituitary adenomas: functional and non-functional
- Craniopharyngiomas
- Meningiomas, gliomas, hamartomas
- Dysgerminomas
- Pinealomas
- Metastases (lung, breast, prostate)
- Lymphoma and plasmacytoma

Vascular

- Pituitary infarction:
  —pituitary apoplexy
  —postpartum necrosis (Sheehan's syndrome)
  —post coronary artery bypass graft
  —sickle cell disease
  —antiphospholipid syndrome
  —snakebite coagulopathy (disseminated intravascular coagulation)
- Giant internal carotid artery aneurysms

Infiltrative and inflammatory

- Lymphocytic hypophysitis (autoimmune, also granulomatous and xanthomatous types)
- Sarcoidosis
- Histiocytosis
- Wegener's granulomatosis
- Haemochromatosis
- Vasculitides (e.g. systemic lupus erythematosus)

Infectious diseases

- Tuberculosis, brucellosis, abscess
- Syphilis, HIV

Traumatic and destructive

- Fracture of base of skull with stalk transection
- Pituitary surgery and/or radiotherapy
- Cranial irradiation for malignancy

Congenital

- Single or multiple hormone deficits (see Table 1.1)

Functional

- Psychosocial deprivation in childhood (GH, LH, FSH)
- Chronic disease states (GH, LH, FSH; TSH, in sick euthyroid)
- Anxiety or depression (LH, FSH)
- Weight loss or low body mass index (LH, FSH)
- Anorexia nervosa (LH, FSH; TSH when severe)
- Athlete's syndrome (LH, FSH)

maturation (Ch. 2). The adult GH deficiency syndrome is due to the multiple effects of reduced GH/IGF-1 secretion on body composition (increased central adiposity and reduced muscle mass), cardiorespiratory function and probably also brain function. In the extreme form, individuals complain of marked weakness, lack of drive or energy, tiredness, depression and social isolation. The full syndrome is analogous to the metabolic syndrome, with hypertension, hyperlipidaemia and insulin resistance. In addition, patients may be osteopenic or osteoporotic. Overall mortality is increased by two- to threefold, probably due to cardiac and cerebrovascular causes. However, it must be emphasized that the clinical features are highly variable between individuals and, because of the non-specificity of the symptoms, the syndrome can be diagnosed only when all other hormone deficiencies are adequately replaced.

LH/FSH deficiency

The hypothalamic–pituitary–gonadal axis is usually the next most sensitive to diseases affecting pituitary function. While premenopausal women present most frequently with altered menstrual function (oligoamenorrhoea) and/or infertility, postmenopausal women and men are most often referred because of the chance findings of secondary biochemical hypogonadism (low or normal LH/FSH) or hypothyroidism, the coincidental finding of a pituitary mass or the mass effects of a pituitary lesion (headache and/or visual loss). Men do not often complain of loss of libido or erectile dysfunction unless this question is addressed specifically since they often assume that any changes are due to normal ageing. Men with secondary hypogonadism may be referred with reduced fertility due to oligoazoospermia or occasionally galactorrhoea and hot flushes but they usually have a normal male hair distribution, shaving frequency and testicular size. The 'classic' hypogonadal features of absent secondary sexual hair, reduced facial hair, pallor, soft/podgy hands and fine perioral skin wrinkling indicate long-standing or congenital hypogonadism (Fig. 1.2). If the hypogonadism occurs prior to epiphyseal fusion with normal GH secretion, there may be excessive linear growth leading to eunuchoidism (span greater than height).

TSH and ACTH deficiency

Secondary hypothyroidism is often very variable in degree, and there may be few clear signs and symptoms (tiredness, weight gain, constipation, mental slowing, dry skin and delayed reflex relaxation). Usually, the thyroid gland is impalpable.

Symptoms of hypoadrenalism are non-specific and include malaise, fatigue, loss of appetite, weight loss, headache and lightheadedness. In contrast to primary adrenal insufficiency, patients are pale rather than pigmented and are not usually hypovolaemic and/or hyperkalaemic (ACTH does not have a major influence on aldosterone secretion), but they may show mild hyponatraemia and postural hypotension.

Alterations in PRL secretion

Prolactin deficiency is extremely uncommon and limited to those with certain forms of congenital hypopituitarism or pituitary infarction (e.g. Sheehan's syndrome). Deficiency causes postpartum failure of lactation. In contrast, disinhibition of PRL release with mild hyperprolactinaemia due to stalk compression is encountered much more frequently in hypopituitarism (see below).

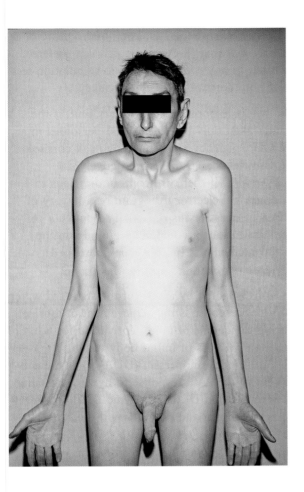

Figure 1.2
A 57-year-old man with long-standing hypopituitarism. Note the sallow complexion and total absence of facial and body hair.

Vasopressin/oxytocin deficiency

Cranial diabetes insipidus (DI) is characterized by polyuria, frequent nocturia and polydipsia. It is seen most commonly with inflammatory, infiltrative or neoplastic lesions or trauma affecting the PP, the pituitary stalk and/or the hypothalamus and is extremely rare in association with disease limited to the AP such as pituitary adenomas. Oxytocin deficiency is not associated with any specific clinical syndromes.

General investigation of hypopituitarism

A full history and thorough examination are necessary to elicit the symptoms and signs of specific trophic hormone deficiencies and the specific endocrinopathies of either functional pituitary adenomas or the many other disorders that can cause hypopituitarism (Box 1.1), and to delineate any possible underlying genetic syndromes. Examination should include visual field testing by confrontation, ideally using a red pin, together with fundoscopy. Basal screening investigations should include measurement of trophic and target gland hormones to distinguish primary and secondary deficiency states for microadenomas and 6-monthly for macroadenomas. However, patients should be warned to make immediate contact should any symptoms develop. Trans-sphenoidal surgery should be undertaken in those with expanding lesions and the presence at presentation or development of neuro-ophthalmological signs (an indication for consideration of urgent surgery).

Serious complications (neural damage, persistent cerebrospinal fluid rhinorrhoea, meningitis) are uncommon following surgery, and mortality should be less than 1%. However, varying degrees of hypopituitarism are not uncommon (occasionally including DI, which recovers in most individuals over a few months), and full reassessment of AP function, including MRI, should be undertaken, usually by 4–6 weeks after surgery.

With the availability of close radiological monitoring, external beam irradiation is now used much more cautiously and less frequently because of the rare problems of visual failure, long-term cerebrovascular effects and possible tumour formation (astrocytoma, glioblastoma, meningioma, sarcoma). However, radiotherapy still has an important place in the treatment of those in whom surgery is contraindicated or when an expanding residual adenoma is inaccessible to further surgery. When used, the dosage should not exceed 4500 rad delivered over 5–6 weeks in at least 25 fractions of no more than 180 rad. The risk of side-effects can be further reduced by using the more focused delivery of gamma knife stereotactic surgery, but as yet this is only available in a few specialized centres. The development of hypopituitarism (GH, then LH/FSH, then ACTH/TSH) following radiotherapy occurs slowly over many years (up to 15–20 years), and at least annual assessment of pituitary function is required with appropriate hormone replacement as and when indicated.

Craniopharyngiomas and other neoplasms

A wide range of other neoplasms, all of them rare, can cause varying degrees and patterns of hypopituitarism. Probably the most common are craniopharyngiomas, which comprise up to 5% of intracranial neoplasms. They are benign and derived from the vestigial remnants of Rathke's pouch epithelium. The so-called adamantinomatous type (usually cystic, intrasellar with or without suprasellar extension, and calcified) present during the first two decades, whereas the less frequent papillary variety (solid and usually suprasellar or third ventricular) usually present in the fourth decade. Both varieties can present with visual loss, variable hypopituitarism, stalk compression hyperprolactinaemia, hydrocephalus in children and raised intracranial pressure in adults, with associated mental disturbance and DI in 15–30%. Complete surgical resection is curative, but troublesome recurrences are not uncommon following incomplete resection. The role of radiotherapy is controversial.

Dysgerminomas are extremely rare germ cell tumours usually occurring in childhood and young adulthood. Recognition is important, because they respond extremely well to combined radiotherapy and chemotherapy. They can present with variable hypopituitarism, stalk compression hyperprolactinaemia, DI and/or mass effects. The diagnosis, while supported by the finding of elevated serum and/or cerebrospinal fluid β-human chorionic gonadotrophin levels, ultimately depends on biopsy.

Vascular causes

Variable degrees of haemorrhage into pre-existing adenomas are probably quite common although usually clinically silent, revealed only by MRI. Headache may be associated with these minor episodes, but the clinical syndrome of apoplexy with sudden onset of severe headache is much less common. In its severest form, apoplexy can present with complete pituitary infarction and/or variable degrees of visual loss or ophthalmoplegia. The presentation can mimic that of subarachnoid haemorrhage and apoplexy must be considered in the differential diagnosis of severe intracranial haemorrhage. Important practical points are that adequate examination of the drowsy or comatose patient may reveals signs of hypopituitarism, and requests for emergency CT should include adequate views of the hypothalamic–pituitary region. Parenteral glucocorticoids should be administered urgently if there is any clinical suspicion of this diagnosis.

With improvements in obstetric care, pituitary infarction secondary to postpartum haemorrhage (Sheehan's syndrome) is uncommon in western society and is usually seen among immigrants from poorer countries. The classic picture is failure of lactation and persistent secondary amenorrhoea, but both the degree and pattern of hypopituitarism can be quite variable.

There are a variety of case reports describing the occurrence of pituitary infarction and anterior hypopituitarism in association with blood volume or flow manipulation (coronary artery bypass graft), coagulopathies including disseminated intravascular coagulation, and vasculitides (e.g. systemic lupus erythematosus).

Finally, giant internal carotid artery aneurysms can occasionally mimic macroadenomas, but recognition of these is now straightforward with MRI, which should always be undertaken prior to any pituitary surgery.

Infiltrative and inflammatory causes

Hypopituitarism can occur occasionally in association with a wide range of inflammatory, granulomatous and infiltrative conditions. Probably the commonest encountered are lymphocytic hypophysitis and sarcoidosis.

Lymphocytic hypophysitis is believed to be an autoimmune condition, because it often occurs in association with other autoimmune diseases and is seen most often in late pregnancy or the early postpartum period. However, it can occur outside this setting and has also been reported in males. Once again, it can present with variable degrees of hypopituitarism, stalk compression hyperprolactinaemia and/or DI. ACTH deficiency is commonest and may be the only problem in milder forms. Quite often, it is a benign, self-limiting condition and hypopituitarism may improve, but occasionally mass effects can develop (particularly visual failure) and hypopituitarism remain fixed. Hypopituitarism should be treated and close radiological monitoring undertaken. If there is progression, steroid therapy is beneficial in some and should be tried prior to consideration of debulking surgery.

The non-caseating granulomas of sarcoidosis can infiltrate any part of the hypothalamic–pituitary unit, either in isolation or as part of more widespread neurosarcoidosis. Such involvement is said to occur in up to 5% of patients with systemic disease. Once again, hypopituitarism and stalk compression hyperprolactinaemia can be variable in degree, and DI or mass effects may be the presenting feature. Firm diagnosis of isolated hypothalamic–pituitary disease depends on biopsy but plasma or cerebrospinal fluid angiotensin-converting enzyme levels can be helpful. In progressive disease, glucocorticoid therapy is usually undertaken, with or without immunosuppressive therapy.

Although MRI can help to distinguish many intrasellar, pituitary stalk, suprasellar and parasellar lesions, ultimately biopsy may be necessary to determine the precise diagnosis and appropriate management. Prior to this, examination of the cerebrospinal fluid for α-fetoprotein, β-human chorionic gonadotrophin and angiotensin-converting enzyme levels should be undertaken.

Congenital causes

Knowledge of the specific gene mutations underlying various rare types of congenital hypopituitarism has advanced rapidly in recent years (Table 1.1), but clinical management remains the same with respect to appropriate hormone replacement therapy.

Table 1.1: Causes of congenital hypopituitarism

	Deficiency	Phenotype	Gene mutation
Single	GH	Short stature	GH-1, GHRH-R
	TSH	Hypothyroidism	TSH-β, TRH-R
	LH/FSH	Hypogonadotrophic hypogonadism	LH-β, FSH-β, GnRH-R
		• with anosmia, synkinesis, renal agenesis (Kallmann's syndrome type 1)	KAL-1
		• with anosmia, cleft lip or palate (Kallmann's syndrome type 2)	FGFR-1
		• with sex reversal or adrenal failure	SF-1
		• with adrenal hypoplasia	DAX-1
		• with obesity	Leptin, leptin-R
	ACTH	Hypoadrenalism	TPIT
		• with obesity, red hair	POMC
	AVP	Familial diabetes insipidus	AVP–neurophysin-2
Multiple	GH, TSH, LH/FSH, ACTH	Anterior hypopituitarism	PROP-1
	GH, PRL, TSH	Partial hypopituitarism	PIT-1
	GH plus several	Partial hypopituitarism, septo-optic dysplasia	HESX-1
	GH, PRL, TSH, LH/FSH	Partial hypopituitarism	LHX-3
	GH, TSH, ACTH	Partial hypopituitarism	LHX-4

(After Drouin J et al. 2006 In: Ho K, Chihara K (eds) Molecular pathogenesis and therapy of pituitary disease. Bioscientifica, Bristol, pp. 1–10, with permission.)

Most forms of congenital hypopituitarism should be detected soon after birth (because of ill health or failure to thrive) or during infancy and childhood (growth retardation). The exception is hypogonadotrophic hypogonadism due to Kallmann's syndrome, which may not be recognized until adolescence (delayed pubertal development) or adulthood (hypogonadism and/or infertility).

Kallmann's syndrome describes hypogonadotrophic hypogonadism due to GnRH deficiency (failure of migration of GnRH neurons during embryogenesis), with hyposmia or anosmia due to underdevelopment of olfactory tissue. It is around five times more frequent in males and is heterogeneous, both genetically and phenotypically. Familial cases indicate X chromosome-linked, autosomal dominant and occasional recessive forms of inheritance, but most cases are sporadic and incomplete penetrance may be significant so that both hypogonadism and olfactory problems can vary markedly, even within an affected family. Kallmann's type 1 (X chromosome linked) is due to KAL-1 gene mutations and has the additional clinical features of mirror movements (bimanual synkinesis in 75%) and renal agenesis (30%). Type 2 (autosomal dominant) is due to mutations in the fibroblast growth factor receptor type 1 (FGFR-1), and cleft lip or palate is common but mirror movements are rare. Overall, only 20% of patients have KAL-1 or FGFR-1 mutations, so the others remain to be elucidated.

Functional causes

These most commonly affect GH and gonadotrophin secretion and in many cases reflect the body's physiological response to a variety of external stresses or chronic disease states. Psychosocial deprivation or chronic disease in childhood causes GH and gonadotrophin deficiency, with consequent growth retardation and delayed pubertal development.

Severe stress and weight loss with low body mass index (BMI) can cause both primary and secondary amenorrhoea, or low testosterone levels in males due to hypogonadotrophic hypogonadism, as typified in the extreme form, anorexia nervosa. In the so-called athlete's syndrome, low BMI and a rigorous exercise schedule can cause hypogonadotrophic hypogonadism in both males and females. Severe acute and chronic disease states can each cause hypogonadotrophic hypogonadism and central TSH suppression (low or low normal basal TSH levels with reduced free T_4 – the so-called euthyroid sick syndrome).

Although all these responses reflect the body's attempt to conserve energy in the face of demanding situations, if the hypogonadism is prolonged it can lead to osteopenia or osteoporosis and is a not infrequent cause of reduced fertility in both men and women.

Treatment of hypopituitarism

The treatment of specific hormone deficiencies is relatively straightforward, but two particular points must be borne in mind.

- Glucocorticoid replacement should be commenced for at least a few days before thyroid hormone replacement, because T_4 can precipitate adrenal crisis in glucocorticoid-deficient patients.
- GH replacement should not be commenced until all other hormone replacement deficiencies are adequately treated.

Glucocorticoid replacement

Although the standard approach has been to use hydrocortisone, trying to mimic the circadian variation in cortisol secretion, dosage regimens do vary considerably. Most patients are perfectly well on 10 mg b.d. regimens, but an initial dose of 15 mg on waking and 5 mg around 6 p.m. is often tried. Replacement should be adjusted to as low a dose as possible, and a total daily dose of 15 mg can be achieved in some. Complaints of afternoon tiredness and malaise can be alleviated sometimes by splitting the total daily dose so that it is taken on waking, at lunchtime and in the evening. Finally, patients should be advised to:

- double or triple their daily dose during episodes of severe stress or intercurrent illness
- carry a steroid replacement card
- wear a necklace or bracelet indicating that they are taking glucocorticoid replacement therapy.

Thyroid hormone replacement

Thyroxine is usually given at an average daily dose of between 100 and 200 µg daily. Because the TSH level is of no monitoring value in hypopituitarism, the T_4 dosage should be titrated against the patient's symptoms, aiming for free triiodothyronine and free T_4 levels in the mid to upper normal range. In elderly patients, it is prudent to start replacement with 25–50 µg, gradually increasing as required.

Gonadal hormone replacement

Gonadal hormone replacement is important, even in asymptomatic individuals, to protect against bone loss and the long-term development of osteoporosis and probably also vascular disease in both men and women. In women, it is best achieved with a conventional oral contraceptive preparation providing that there are no contraindications. Alternatively, there are a range of preparations for continuous oestrogen and progesterone administration to avoid withdrawal bleeding in women who prefer this. Women who have undergone hysterectomy require oestrogen replacement only. A more physiological approach preferred by some is to use transdermal preparations, which are reported to maintain oestradiol levels in the physiological range. However, the contraceptive value of these formulations has not been established.

In men, the standard approach has been to use intramuscular injections of testosterone enantate or propionate every 2–4 weeks, but this also has been superseded by transdermal preparations in the form of patches or gels, long-acting injections (testosterone undecanoate) or buccal tablets, which provide more stable physiological testosterone levels. In older men (>50 years), it is prudent to check the prostate and prostate-specific antigen levels prior to commencement and annually thereafter.

GH replacement

GH replacement must be administered according to National Institute for Health and Clinical Excellence guidelines based on quality of life issues rather than any potential long-term vascular benefits that are not yet established. Patients must score above 11 in the quality of life rating scale (assessment of GH deficiency in adults score) and show an improvement of at least 7 points during a 9-month therapeutic trial. The replacement dose is titrated against the IGF-1 level, aiming for a value in the upper normal range, with monitoring of BMI, blood pressure, fasting glucose and lipids. With the low doses of GH that are generally required, the side-effects of excess GH (oedema, hypertension, carpal tunnel syndrome and carbohydrate intolerance) found in early studies are very uncommon.

AVP replacement

Arginine vasopressin replacement is undertaken using an AVP analogue, desmopressin acetate (DDAVP), which is usually administered intranasally at a dosage of either 10 μg daily or b.d. Precise dosage and frequency can be adjusted according to the patient's symptoms, and occasional monitoring of the urea and electrolytes can be helpful because the development of hyponatraemia indicates probable overtreatment. An oral preparation of DDAVP is available for those who wish to try this, but in practice it is used much less commonly than the intranasal preparation.

HYPERPROLACTINAEMIA

Hyperprolactinaemia is the commonest pituitary disorder that we encounter, and prolactinomas are the commonest type of pituitary adenoma (seen most frequently in women). There is a wide range of possible causes of sustained hyperprolactinaemia (Box 1.2) that must be considered before reaching a diagnosis of a primary pituitary disturbance in PRL control mechanisms.

The most frequent causes are pregnancy and drugs that reduce the synthesis or action of DA on lactotrophs. Although the combined oral contraceptive may cause a slight elevation in PRL levels due to the oestrogen component, these drugs do not cause significant, sustained hyperprolactinaemia (as compared with the much higher doses of oestrogen that used to be used in some forms of hormone replacement therapy). Several other diseases can cause significant, non-adenomatous hyperprolactinaemia, the most relevant being:

- primary hypothyroidism (possibly due to reduced DA_2 receptor activity and/or increased TRH action on lactotrophs)
- polycystic ovarian syndrome (PCOS; increased oestrogenic stimulation of lactotrophs)
- severe chronic renal/liver disease (precise causes unknown).

Box 1.2: Causes of sustained hyperprolactinaemia

- Pregnancy
- Chronic nipple stimulation, chest wall surgery, trauma (afferent nerve stimulation)
- Drugs:
  —dopamine depletors – methyldopa, monoamine oxidase inhibitors (pargyline), DA_2 receptor antagonists (metoclopramide, domperidone, phenothiazines and the atypical antipsychotics risperidone and molindone) and the tricyclic antidepressant clomipramine[a]
  —oestrogens (only in high dosage; not usually seen with low-dose oral contraceptives or transdermal preparations)
- Primary hypothyroidism (10–20%)
- Polycystic ovarian syndrome (20–30%)
- Chronic renal failure (including haemodialysis)
- Chronic liver disease
- Stalk compression hyperprolactinaemia (all causes of hypopituitarism in Box 1.1 except pituitary infarction, specific types of congenital hypopituitarism and functional causes; NFPAs are the commonest in practice)
- Prolactinomas (including mixed secretory tumours: GH/PRL and ACTH/PRL)
- Idiopathic (but many probably have microprolactinomas beyond the resolution of computerized tomography or magnetic resonance imaging)

[a]Occasionally, amitryptiline, desipramine, quetiapine and olanzapine may cause mild hyperprolactinaemia, but by and large selective serotonin reuptake inhibitors do not cause this problem.

When pregnancy, drugs and other diseases have been excluded, consideration should be given as to whether the hyperprolactinaemia is caused by any disease process reducing the synthesis and transport of DA to the AP (thus enabling disinhibition of lactotrophs) or to a prolactinoma. In broad terms, this includes virtually all the conditions that may cause hypopituitarism listed in Box 1.1, with the exception of pituitary infarction (low or undetectable PRL levels), specific congenital hormone deficiencies and functional causes. In practice, the most frequent causes of so-called stalk compression hyperprolactinaemia are pituitary macroadenomas, both non-functional and functional.

Clinical features

Sustained hyperprolactinaemia from any cause leads to hypogonadotrophic hypogonadism due to suppression of the normal pulsatile release of LH and FSH, as well as through direct antagonism of their gonadal actions. Women are usually referred with oligoamenorrhoea with or without galactorrhoea and/or reduced fertility. Men usually present much later than women (unless referred because of the finding of oligoazoospermia during investigation for infertility), because they do not often complain about reduced libido or potency, attributing this to normal ageing or other factors. In consequence, men present most often with macroprolactinomas causing more extensive hypopituitarism and/or neuro-ophthalmological problems due to mass effects. Unlike in women, galactorrhoea is extremely uncommon but is pathognomonic of hyperprolactinaemia when present.

Investigation

Guidelines for the investigation and management of hyperprolactinaemia have been published recently under the auspices of the International Pituitary Society. A full history and examination should readily exclude drug effects and other relevant disease states, supported by appropriate investigations (Box 1.3). It should be remembered, however, that primary hypothyroidism and PCOS are common and may coexist in patients with prolactinomas. Many relatively asymptomatic patients are referred with only marginally elevated PRL levels that may well be due to the stress of venepuncture, because levels are often normal on repeat testing in less stressful, resting conditions.

Caution may sometimes be required in the interpretation of raised PRL levels. Depending on the type of assay used, 'raised' levels may be due to the presence of biologically and clinically irrelevant 'macroprolactin' (large aggregates of the PRL molecule) but this is usually routinely excluded in the laboratory using polyethylene glycol precipitation. Exceptionally high PRL levels due to macroprolactinomas can sometimes interfere in immunoradiometric assays, giving lower than expected results (the 'high dose hook' effect). However, this can be checked easily using serial dilutions and is rarely a clinical problem.

Some centres find that dynamic assessment of the TSH and PRL responses to acute DA receptor blockade (10 mg of domperidone intravenously with samples for TSH and PRL at 0′ and 30′) is helpful in the diagnosis of microprolactinoma. Characteristically, patients with microprolactinomas show exaggerated TSH and reduced PRL release following such acute DA disinhibition, whereas a normal pattern of response is seen in those with PCOS or macroprolactinaemia.

Prolactin levels greater than 5000 mU/L are virtually diagnostic of a prolactinoma, whereas levels lower than this could be due to either a prolactinoma or to stalk compression from another lesion. When all other causes have been excluded, most patients with sustained hyperprolactinaemia will prove to have a microadenoma on CT or MRI. When imaging is normal, the label idiopathic hyperprolactinaemia is sometimes used, but it seems likely that many such individuals harbour microprolactinomas beyond the resolution of CT or MRI.

Box 1.3: Investigation of hyperprolactinaemia

- Basal, resting PRL levels
- Pregnancy test
- Oestradiol or testosterone, LH, FSH
- Free thyroxine, TSH
- Urea and electrolytes, liver function tests (but chronic disease will usually be obvious)
- Testosterone, dehydroepiandrosterone sulphate, androstenedione and transvaginal ovarian ultrasound (if indicated by history and signs)
- Dual energy x-ray absorptiometry (if evidence of long-standing hypogonadism)
- Pituitary computerized tomography or magnetic resonance imaging if hyperprolactinaemia confirmed
- No further investigation if microadenoma (<10 mm)
- Full assessment of AP function (including insulin stress test if no contraindication) if macroadenoma (>10 mm)

Management

If relevant and possible, drug withdrawal should be undertaken for 2–3 days to check whether PRL levels are normalized. If not possible or levels remain high and the patient is euthyroid, then CT/MRI should be undertaken. Elevated PRL levels due to primary hypothyroidism are normalized by adequate T$_4$ replacement, usually within 3 months.

When required, the treatment of choice for idiopathic hyperprolactinaemia and prolactinomas of all sizes is medical therapy with DA agonist drugs. Several such drugs have been developed, but in practice most patients can be treated very effectively with either bromocriptine (the parent compound) or cabergoline. Cabergoline is preferred, because it is more potent and longer acting (it need only be taken once or twice weekly by mouth) than bromocriptine, with fewer side-effects. However, all DA agonists share a similar side-effect profile, with nausea, vomiting and postural hypotension, but these are usually mild, improve over the first couple of weeks of treatment, and are minimized by building up the dosage gradually. DA agonist therapy restores normal PRL levels, gonadal function and fertility in the vast majority of women and men with idiopathic hyperprolactinaemia or microprolactinomas. Additionally, it causes prolactinoma shrinkage (both micro and macro) of at least 25% in 80–90% within 12 months (Fig. 1.4).

Hyperprolactinaemia with normal CT/MRI or microadenoma

Not all women require DA agonist therapy unless fertility is wanted, although some prefer this therapeutic option. All those in whom DA agonists are used should be warned that fertility is often restored rapidly (sometimes before the restoration of menses), and appropriate precautions should be taken if conception is not desired. If restoration of fertility is the primary aim, treatment with bromocriptine is preferred, because more safety data are available for this drug (no evidence of increased foetal malformations or perinatal problems) compared with cabergoline. Women should be advised to wait until

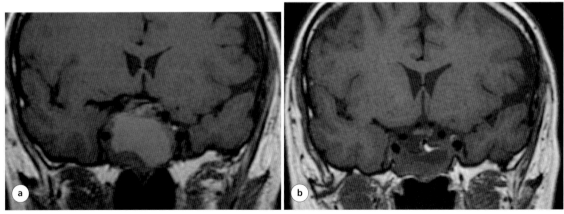

Figure 1.4
Dramatic shrinkage of a macroprolactinoma **(a)** before and **(b)** after commencing cabergoline 0.5 mg twice weekly. This 29-year-old man presented with bitemporal hemianopia, which resolved completely within 12 h of his first dose of cabergoline. His pretreatment prolactin was 85 000 mU/L, which was normalized by 6 months of treatment. Although his gonadal function improved, he requires ongoing testosterone supplementation.

Box 1.4: Management of hyperprolactinaemia with normal CT/MRI or microadenoma

- Asymptomatic women (more than six menses/year, no troublesome galactorrhoea):
  —no absolute need for dopamine agonist, but monitor with annual PRL and CT/MRI if indicated
  —no contraindication to use of oral contraceptives (no evidence of increased adenoma size)
- Symptomatic women (fewer than six menses/year, low oestradiol, troublesome galactorrhoea):
  —hormone replacement therapy using oral contraceptives alone is safe if fertility not required
  —annual PRL with CT/MRI if indicated
  —alternatively, cabergoline (increasing to 0.5 mg once or twice weekly) can be used if there is troublesome galactorrhoea, along with oral contraceptives if conception not wanted
  —if fertility wanted, use bromocriptine, increasing to 2.5 mg b.d. or t.i.d.
- Symptomatic men (loss of libido, impotence, low testosterone and/or oligospermia):
  —use cabergoline, increasing to 0.5 mg once or twice weekly

---

restoration of menses before trying to conceive, and then to stop treatment and check a pregnancy test if a period is missed. A suggested approach is outlined in Box 1.4.

Most microprolactinomas (90–95%) do not enlarge, but under the high oestrogen drive of pregnancy, clinically significant expansion can occur in up to 2%. Monitoring is important therefore, and women must be warned to make contact in the event of a severe headache or visual disturbance. If MRI shows significant adenoma expansion, reintroduction of DA agonist therapy will usually re-establish control and surgery is required only rarely.

Hyperprolactinaemia with macroadenoma but no mass effects

The management of hyperprolactinaemia with a macroadenoma raises different issues, particularly if the PRL level is less than 5000 mU/L, which might be due to stalk compression. A suggested approach is outlined in Box 1.5.

Box 1.5: Management of hyperprolactinaemia with macroadenoma and no mass effects

- Full assessment of AP function with IST or GH-releasing hormone/arginine and short synacthen test
  —Treat hypopituitarism but withhold gonadal replacement until response to dopamine (DA) agonist therapy is determined
- Prolactin (PRL) >5000 mU/L: diagnosis is prolactinoma
  —Use cabergoline, increasing to 0.5 mg once or twice weekly
- PRL <5000 mU/L: may be stalk compression from NFPA, other lesion or prolactinoma
  —Trial of cabergoline (even in those with atypical neuroradiological features), with repeat CT/MRI at 3 months
  —If adenoma shrinks, the likely diagnosis is prolactinoma, so continue therapy (PRL response is non-specific, because DA agonists will normalize elevated PRL levels from any cause)
  —If no shrinkage and PRL normal, continue therapy and repeat CT/MRI in 6 months (shrinkage occurs slowly in some prolactinomas); if increase in size, consider surgery for removal and/or biopsy
- Initial PRL only marginally elevated (550–1000 mU/L): most likely stalk compression
  —DA agonist unlikely to benefit
  —Monitoring (CT/MRI), treatment of hypopituitarism and treatment of adenoma if close to chiasm

Women with macroprolactinomas who wish to conceive should plan for this after PRL is normalized and significant shrinkage has occurred. Furthermore, because clinically relevant adenoma expansion can occur in up to 20–30%, the continuation of DA agonist therapy throughout pregnancy is justifiable, although not all use this approach but reintroduce DA agonists if there is clinical and MRI evidence of expansion.

Hyperprolactinaemia with macroadenoma and mass effects

This is usually urgent and in some cases an emergency situation. An approach to management is outlined in Box 1.6.

When DA agonist therapy is used for a suspected macroprolactinoma in a hypogonadal patient, gonadal replacement should be commenced if there is no return of function following normalization of PRL levels, because pituitary function may have been irreversibly destroyed.

Dopamine agonist withdrawal, resistance and intolerance

Consideration should be given to DA agonist reduction and withdrawal every 2–3 years if the PRL level has been normalized and there is significant adenoma shrinkage. Recent evidence indicates that remission may be achieved in perhaps 30% for at least 2 years. Close follow-up is necessary, particularly for previous macroadenomas, with monitoring of PRL levels and further radiology if indicated.

Up to 10–20% of patients may show some degree of DA agonist resistance or intolerance. Other DA agonists (pergolide, quinagolide) can be tried, but if this is unhelpful trans-sphenoidal surgery may be considered (but only in experienced centres). The results for microprolactinoma surgery are good, with cure rates varying from 75 to 90% and, despite a variably reported recurrence rate (up to 20% within 5 years), a few patients prefer the surgical approach to long-term DA agonist treatment. Not surprisingly, the surgical success rate for cure of macroprolactinomas is markedly less.

Box 1.6: Management of hyperprolactinaemia with macroadenoma and mass effects

- Full assessment of AP status including urgent PRL/cortisol (short synacthen or IST if possible)
  —Treat hypopituitarism
  —Withhold gonadal replacement until DA agonist response is determined
- PRL >5000 mU/L: diagnostic of prolactinoma (levels usually in the tens or hundreds of thousands)
  —Use cabergoline (0.5 mg) with close monitoring; macroprolactinomas usually show rapid (12–24 h) improvement in visual fields or acuity (and other mass effects) with rapid fall in PRL
  —If no improvement after 48 h or if deterioration occurs, consider urgent surgery
  —If improvement, continue cabergoline (0.5 mg twice weekly) and repeat PRL/MRI at 3 months
  —Continue dose titration of cabergoline to normalize PRL levels
- Initial PRL only marginally elevated (550–1000 mU/L): probably stalk compression due to NFPA or other lesion
  —Consider urgent surgery

ACROMEGALY

This is a rare condition (around two or three cases/million per year) due, in almost all cases, to a pituitary somatotroph adenoma. Most cases are sporadic, but occasional familial occurrences have been described. Somatotroph hyperplasia due to ectopic GHRH production (most commonly by a bronchial carcinoid tumour or pancreatic neuroendocrine tumour, but also reported in association with small cell carcinoma of the lung, adrenal adenomas, phaeochromocytomas and hypothalamic hamartomas or gliomas) is extremely rare (<1%), and there has only been one reported case (although well documented) of ectopic GH production by a pancreatic endocrine tumour. Somatotroph adenomas also occur rarely as part of the multiple endocrine neoplasia type 1 syndrome and in association with other rare endocrine tumour syndromes such as the McCune–Albright syndrome and Carney complex (see Table 1.2 and Ch. 9).

Most somatotroph adenomas (about 60%) secrete GH only, but co-secretion of PRL also occurs, either from two cell types (25%) or from a single-cell mammosomatotroph adenoma (10%). Hyperprolactinaemia may also be due to stalk compression by a macroadenoma. Hypersecretion of other hormones (ACTH, TSH and α subunit) may also be encountered occasionally.

Clinical features

GH and IGF-1 exert widespread effects, and chronic exposure to excess levels causes marked morbidity and premature mortality (perhaps by up to 10 years), due mainly to cardiovascular and cerebrovascular problems (Box 1.7). There is also an increased risk of malignancy (particularly carcinoma of colon and probably also breast) in untreated acromegaly, and premalignant colonic polyps are not uncommon (more frequently found in patients with skin tags). This is in keeping with recent epidemiological evidence from the normal population, which shows a positive correlation between IGF-1 levels and the incidence of various malignancies (colon, breast, prostate and lung).

Because the clinical features develop slowly over many years, acromegaly can remain unrecognized until quite late in the disease process. However, due to increased awareness and earlier diagnosis, the classic clinical features of acromegaly (coarse facial features, prognathism, dental malocclusion, thick greasy skin, and broad spade-like hands and feet) are seen less frequently. The important point is that investigation should be undertaken even if there is only a slight suspicion of acromegaly, despite the absence of some or all of the classic features, because earlier diagnosis and treatment lead to better outcomes (Fig. 1.5).

Investigation

Diagnosis depends on the demonstration of a lack of suppression of GH levels to less than 0.5 mU/L (using current high-sensitivity assays) in response to 75 g of oral glucose

---

Box 1.7: Long-term effects of excess GH and IGF-1 levels

Skin and soft tissues

- Thick, greasy skin, increased sweating (very common)
- Increased skin tags
- Soft tissue enlargement; increased size of hands and feet
- Coarse facial features, with frontal prominence, prognathism and dental malocclusion

Musculoskeletal

- Tall stature or gigantism if prior to epiphyseal fusion
- Arthralgias
- Degenerative osteoarthrosis
- Proximal muscle weakness

Nervous system

- Frontal headache (very common)
- Varied compressive mononeuropathies (especially carpal tunnel syndrome)
- Sensorimotor neuropathy

Cardiorespiratory system

- Hypertension and ischaemic heart disease
- Specific cardiomyopathy (left ventricular or septal hypertrophy, diastolic dysfunction, dysrhythmias) leading to congestive heart failure
- Upper airways obstruction (soft tissue enlargement)
- Sleep apnoea syndrome

Metabolic and endocrine

- Insulin resistance with hyperlipidaemia
- Carbohydrate intolerance or frank diabetes, especially if familial hypercholesterolaemia
- Hypercalciuria
- Mild hyperthyroidism due to autonomous nodular goitre

(standard glucose tolerance test), together with elevated, age-related IGF-1 levels. Some patients may show a paradoxical GH rise in response to TRH administration when compared with normal subjects, but this test is rarely required nowadays. GH levels may be elevated and non-suppressible in poorly controlled diabetes, but IGF-1 levels are usually low in this situation. In patients with severe, long-standing disease and hypertension, full evaluation of cardiovascular status should be undertaken, including echocardiography to assess any degree of impairment in left ventricular function. PRL levels may be elevated and mild hyperthyroidism is sometimes present in association with a multinodular goitre. When the diagnosis is confirmed, MRI will reveal a pituitary adenoma in most cases (microadenoma in 25–35%), and normal radiology raises the possibility of an ectopic GHRH source (although there may be minor pituitary enlargement due simply to somatotroph hyperplasia).

Management

In elderly patients with extensive comorbidity, it may well be appropriate to manage the situation conservatively, but hypertension, heart failure and diabetes should be treated

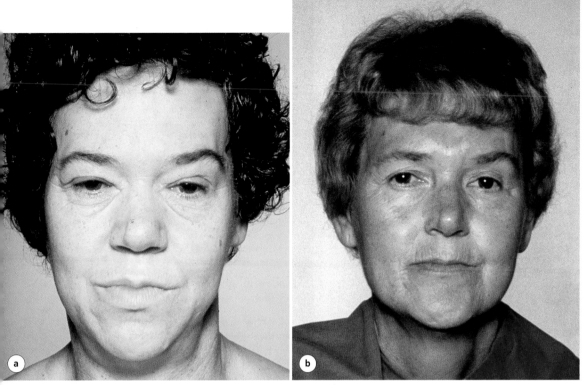

Figure 1.5
Facial appearance **(a)** before and **(b)** 6 years after curative trans-sphenoidal surgery for acromegaly. The mild acromegalic features improved slowly, but the patient's quality of life was destroyed by severe postoperative GH deficiency. She showed a remarkable and dramatic improvement in quality of life when she eventually went on to receive GH replacement therapy.

appropriately when necessary (management of the last of these can be difficult due to insulin resistance). The aim of treatment is to normalize GH and IGF-1 levels while at the same time restoring and/or maintaining normal pituitary function. Current evidence suggests that restoration of GH levels to less than 5 mU/L throughout the day and normalization of IGF-1 reverse increased risk and restore mortality to normal. Approaches to specific treatment include surgery, radiotherapy and medical management.

Surgery

Trans-sphenoidal surgery is the treatment of choice in most patients with somatotroph adenomas. This should be undertaken only by an experienced surgeon in selected centres that deal with a sufficient number of patients to maintain skills. Not surprisingly, the smaller the adenoma and the lower the GH level, the better the outcome, with an expected cure rate of around 80% for microadenomas but only around 40–50% for macroadenomas. Long-term recurrence has been reported in up to 10% of patients despite restoration of GH levels to less than 5 mU/L, probably because of residual adenoma. Successful surgery is followed by rapid symptomatic improvement in headache, sweating and the consequences of soft tissue swelling (e.g. carpal tunnel syndrome, sleep apnoea). IGF-1 levels are usually normalized within a week but may decline over several months in a few, and varying degrees of postoperative hypopituitarism may occur in 15–20%.

Radiotherapy

Conventional external beam irradiation (or gamma knife stereotactic surgery if available) should be considered when surgery is contraindicated or not curative. The same dosages, conditions and side-effects apply as described previously for its use in NFPAs. Unfortunately, however, excess GH secretion declines only very slowly over many years (sometimes up to 20), and hypopituitarism gradually develops over about the same time period.

Medical therapy

DA agonists such as bromocriptine and cabergoline cause a variable decline in circulating GH levels in acromegaly (as compared with the acute GH-releasing effects in normal subjects), but higher and more frequent doses are required than in the treatment of hyperprolactinaemia, and IGF-1 levels are normalized only infrequently (<5%). Despite this, rapid symptomatic improvement (headaches, sweating and soft tissue swelling) can occur in some, and occasional patients can show dramatic biochemical normalization, tumour shrinkage and clinical improvement, especially those with significant hyperprolactinaemia (likely to be mammosomatotroph adenomas). Because it is relatively cheap, a therapeutic trial of DA agonist is certainly worth considering on cost–benefit grounds in those in whom surgery is ineffective or non-curative, and this should certainly be tried as first-line therapy in those with significant hyperprolactinaemia and relatively mild acromegaly.

Long-acting somatostatin analogues (octreotide LAR or lanreotide Autogel) that bind predominantly to somatostatin receptor types 2 and 5, given by monthly injection, are much more effective inhibitors of GH secretion than DA agonists but also much more expensive (e.g. average dosage around £11 000 a year versus £300 a year for cabergoline). In general, the smaller the adenoma and the lower the GH level (also applicable to residual adenoma after debulking macroadenoma surgery), the better the response, and most patients with microadenomas can expect to achieve GH levels less than 5 mU/L with normalization of IGF-1. Although in principle such agents can be tried as first-line therapy, current policy (on cost–benefit grounds) is to use them when surgery is contraindicated or non-curative or while awaiting the beneficial effects of radiotherapy. Mild side-effects are not uncommon and include nausea, colicky abdominal discomfort or pain, mild steatorrhoea (due to fat malabsorption) and flatulence. These usually improve after a few weeks' continued treatment, but occasional individuals are intolerant. A 2-week trial of short-acting subcutaneous octreotide is recommended to assess tolerability prior to commencing depot preparations. In the longer term, 30–40% develop asymptomatic gallstones or biliary sludge, but this is rarely a clinical problem.

Most recently, a specific GH receptor antagonist molecule (pegvisomant) has been approved for use in acromegaly. It is extremely effective in normalizing IGF-1 levels and inducing marked symptomatic relief. There has been concern about possible long-term effects on adenoma size, but most data thus far are reassuring. Unfortunately, it is extremely expensive (and prohibitively so in some regions) at upwards of £20 000 a year, and its use is likely to be limited to the very few patients whose condition is not adequately controlled by a combination of all the above measures.

CUSHING'S DISEASE

In practice, the commonest cause of many of the features of Cushing's syndrome is the use of pharmacological doses of glucocorticoids in the treatment of other disease states (including sometimes the use of potent glucocorticoid inhalers or topical creams). Endogenous Cushing's syndrome is extremely rare (one or two/million per year) and is commoner in women, although we have certainly noticed an increasing number of cases in recent years, probably due to increased diagnostic awareness (e.g. Cushing's syndrome has been reported in up to 4% of obese patients with difficult-to-control type 2 diabetes). Cushing's disease is the term used to describe Cushing's syndrome due to an ACTH-secreting pituitary corticotroph adenoma and is by far the commonest of the several causes of endogenous hypercortisolism (Table 1.2).

Clinical features

Hypersecretion of ACTH causes bilateral adrenal hyperplasia (although this is not always evident radiologically) and hypercortisolism, with many and varied tissue effects.

Table 1.2: Causes of endogenous Cushing's syndrome

Cause	Cases
ACTH-dependent	80–90%
Corticotroph adenoma	75%
Corticotroph hyperplasia	5%
Ectopic ACTH[a]	20%
Ectopic corticotrophin-releasing hormone	Rare
ACTH-independent	10–20%
Adrenal adenoma[b]	60%
Adrenal carcinoma[c]	40%

[a]Usually malignant due to small cell carcinoma of lung but also described with malignancies of pancreas, thymus, ovary, prostate and thyroid (medullary thyroid carcinoma); less commonly benign (bronchial carcinoid, phaeochromocytoma).
[b]Includes unilateral micro- or macronodular disease, ACTH-independent bilateral macronodular adrenal hyperplasia, autonomous adrenal nodule development secondary to pituitary ACTH hypersecretion, McCune–Albright syndrome (Gsα mutation causing polyostotic fibrous dysplasia, pigmented skin lesions, precocious puberty, nodular adrenal hyperplasia, thyroid nodules, acromegaly) and Carney complex (primary pigmented nodular adrenocortical disease, cardiac myxomas, spotty pigmentation of skin, occasionally acromegaly).
[c]Commonest cause of Cushing's syndrome in children younger than 7 years.

Although the clinical features of long-standing disease are well known (Fig. 1.6), not all patients present with these features and the emphasis must be on a high index of suspicion leading to early diagnosis and treatment (Table 1.3). The prognosis of untreated disease is poor, with high morbidity and mortality (up to 50% within 5 years) due mainly to the combined effects of hypertension, diabetes and infection (heart failure, cerebrovascular disease and severe pneumonia, often due to opportunistic infections). Whereas the development of signs and symptoms in primary pituitary disease is relatively slow, hypercortisolism from ectopic ACTH secretion is most commonly due to a malignant process, with the rapid development of weight loss, marked hyperpigmentation (due to very high ACTH levels), severe myopathy and marked metabolic disturbance (hypokalaemic alkalosis). However, patients with ectopic ACTH secretion due to benign

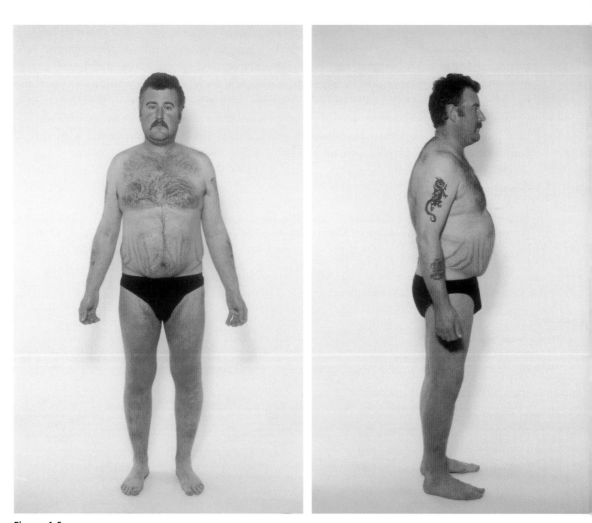

Figure 1.6
A 40-year-old man with classic features of Cushing's syndrome due to an adrenocorticotrophic hormone-secreting pituitary microadenoma: facial plethora, central adiposity, interscapular fat pad (buffalo hump) and pink striae. He was unable to work as a labourer because of severe proximal weakness.

Table 1.3: Clinical features of hypercortisolism (Cushing's syndrome)

Clinical feature	Percentage
Weight gain (central with buffalo hump and moon face)	70–80
Hypertension	70–80
Thin skin with purple striae, easy bruising, plethora	60–70
Mental disturbance (irritability, depression, psychosis)	60–70
Proximal myopathy	50–60
Impotence or oligoamenorrhoea	50–60
Hirsutism and acne	40–70
Osteoporosis (occasionally fractures or vertebral collapse, kyphosis)	40–70
Fluid retention (peripheral or subconjunctival oedema)	30–40
Increased pigmentation (especially ectopic ACTH syndrome)	20–30
Renal stones	<20

causes (e.g. bronchial carcinoid tumours) are often indistinguishable clinically and biochemically from those with Cushing's disease.

Investigation

The procedure is relatively straightforward, but interpretation of the results of investigations must be undertaken cautiously. If there is the slightest clinical suspicion of Cushing's syndrome, we need to ask if hypercortisolism is really present (Box 1.8) and, if so, what is the cause (Box 1.9).

Several other abnormalities are often present in hypercortisolism (Box 1.10) that may help to support the diagnosis if present. Also, it is important to be aware of the varied diagnostic difficulties and pitfalls when interpreting the results of investigations (Box 1.11).

Assessment and management

The initial assessment and management of Cushing's syndrome must include full investigation of metabolic and cardiovascular status. Blood pressure must be controlled and appropriate treatment initiated if there is any evidence of heart failure. Treatment of diabetes mellitus can often be difficult because of the severe insulin resistance. Patients should be screened for any evidence of underlying infection. Successful treatment of hypercortisolism usually leads to rapid improvement in the biochemical, metabolic and psychiatric derangements, although cardiovascular problems may be less responsive, depending on the duration and severity of the disease.

Definitive treatment for Cushing's syndrome depends on the underlying cause. Primary adrenal tumours and ectopic sources of ACTH should be surgically removed, bearing in mind that this may be unachievable and/or inappropriate in the malignant ectopic ACTH syndrome, when palliative chemotherapy and specific adrenal blockade may be all that should be attempted.

Box 1.8: Is hypercortisolism present?

Urinary free cortisol

- High sensitivity (95–100%): false negative with glomerular filtration rate <15 mL/min
- Low specificity: false positive in alcoholism, depression, polycystic ovary syndrome, glucocorticoid resistance (rare)

Overnight dexamethasone suppression

- 1 mg p.o. at midnight followed by 8–9 a.m. plasma cortisol
- High sensitivity (95%) and moderate specificity (85%) with cortisol cut-off <50 nmol/L (ideally, cortisol should be undetectable)
- False positive with oral contraceptive, hormone replacement therapy (oestrogen-induced cortisol-binding globulin elevation) and liver enzyme inducers

Midnight cortisol levels (circadian rhythm)

- Only real value if undetectable sleeping levels, but requires admission
- Late evening, home salivary cortisol may be just as valuable, easier and cheaper

Low-dose dexamethasone suppression

- 0.5 mg q.i.d. for 2 days with 9 a.m. plasma cortisols
- High sensitivity and specificity (98%) with cortisol cut-off <50 nmol/L (ideally, cortisol should be undetectable)
- Sensitivity and specificity enhanced by measuring cortisol response to corticotrophin-releasing factor (100 μg intravenously) at the end (peak cortisol <38 nmol/L in normal subjects); can be useful to distinguish from pseudo-Cushing's syndrome

Insulin stress test

- Absent cortisol response in up to 70% with Cushing's syndrome
- Can be useful to distinguish from pseudo-Cushing's syndrome

Pituitary surgery

Most patients with endogenous hypercortisolism will have Cushing's disease due, in the majority, to an ACTH-secreting pituitary adenoma for which the treatment of choice is trans-sphenoidal surgery undertaken by an experienced surgeon. In the best centres, a remission rate of around 80% can be achieved with minimal hypopituitarism (around 10–20%). With macroadenomas, the results are less good (30–40% remission and a higher rate of hypopituitarism). The optimum result is an undetectable postoperative plasma cortisol level, and such patients will require glucocorticoid replacement therapy (e.g. 1-mg prednisolone tablets; 4 mg a.m./3 mg p.m.) until the suppressed hypothalamic–pituitary–adrenal axis recovers. This can be facilitated by a gradual prednisolone reduction programme (e.g. by 1 mg every 4–6 weeks) until the cortisol response to short synacthen testing is normal. This can take many months and may never be achieved in some individuals, who will require lifelong glucocorticoid replacement therapy. If the postoperative cortisol is greater than 50 nmol/L, further immediate surgery is considered in some centres (up to 5% of patients will have diffuse corticotroph hyperplasia), with the concomitant increased risk of hypopituitarism.

As described previously, full assessment of pituitary function should be undertaken, usually 4–6 weeks postoperatively, and replacement therapy commenced if indicated. It should be remembered that GH deficiency is common in Cushing's disease but often

Box 1.9: What is the cause of hypercortisolism?

Is it ACTH-mediated?

Plasma ACTH level

- Undetectable ACTH confirms primary adrenal hypercortisolism
- Normal or elevated ACTH indicates ACTH-mediated disease
- Low normal ACTH levels usually indicate pituitary source (beware subclinical Cushing's syndrome due to primary adrenal cortical adenoma; see Ch. 5)
- Very high ACTH levels are most probably due to an ectopic source but can also occur with pituitary macroadenomas

Is ACTH-mediated disease pituitary or ectopic?

High-dose dexamethasone suppression

- 2 mg q.i.d. for 2 days with 9 a.m. plasma cortisols
- Cortisol suppression suggests pituitary source, lack of suppression suggests ectopic source, but there is a large overlap
- Therefore relatively low sensitivity (81%) and specificity (67%)

Pituitary neuroradiology

- MRI will detect a microadenoma in most cases of ACTH-mediated disease (but remember the 10% occurrence of pituitary incidentalomas)
- Only around 70% predictive value for lateralization of ACTH-secreting microadenoma

Inferior petrosal sinus sampling with CRH administration

- Central:peripheral ACTH ratio (after CRH) >3 indicates pituitary source
- High sensitivity and specificity (at least 95%), but occasional false positives and negatives reported
- Localization predictive value no better than MRI
- Use judiciously: invasive, labour-intensive, expensive, and occasional vascular and thromboembolic problems have been reported

Additional radiology

- Chest x-ray, CT/MRI of the chest and abdomen if results indicate an ectopic ACTH source
- Octreoscan (radiolabelled somatostatin analogue) will detect ectopic ACTH source in around 50%

Box 1.10: Additional investigations in endogenous hypercortisolism

- Urea and electrolytes: hypokalaemic alkalosis (15–30%)
  —Particularly but not exclusively in malignant ectopic ACTH syndrome
  —impaired renal function if long-standing hypertension or cardiovascular disease
- Full blood count: polycythaemia (up to 20%)
- Thyroid function: often lowish free thyroxine with reduced thyroid-stimulating hormone (TSH; central TSH suppression by increased cortisol levels)
- Hyperprolactinaemia: occasional mixed secretory tumour or stalk compression by macroadenoma
- Hypogonadotrophic hypogonadism (50–60%)
- GH deficiency with low IGF-1: common when looked for in pituitary disease
- Carbohydrate intolerance or diabetes (30–70%)
- Hypercalciuria (up to 20%)
- Osteopenia or osteoporosis (40–70%)

Box 1.11: Causes of diagnostic difficulties in Cushing's syndrome

Drugs

- Oestrogens (oral contraceptive or hormone replacement therapy) raise cortisol-binding globulin and total cortisol
  —False positive overnight or low-dose dexamethasone suppression (stop drugs for 2–3 months prior to test)
  —Urinary free cortisol (UFC) normal
- Anticonvulsants (rifampicin) increase rate of dexamethasone metabolism, causing false positive overnight or low-dose dexamethasone suppression
- Idiosyncratic delay in dexamethasone clearance (rare) can cause false negatives

Pregnancy

- ACTH, cortisol or urinary free cortisol can be raised with reduced dexamethasone suppressibility, particularly in late pregnancy due to placental CRH

Other diseases

- Obesity, PCOS and metabolic syndrome can occasionally be associated with mildly increased UFC, but usually no myopathy and normal overnight or low-dose dexamethasone suppression
- Hyperthyroidism: cortisol-binding globulin and total cortisol may be increased, UFC normal
- Renal impairment: UFC may be low or undetectable if glomerular filtration rate <15 mL/min
- Glucocorticoid resistance (very rare)
  —Glucocorticoid receptor mutations
  —May be asymptomatic or present with hyperandrogenism or hypertension/hypokalaemia
  —Increased cortisol or UFC with reduced dexamethasone suppressibility, but normal circadian rhythm and cortisol response to IST

Pseudo-Cushing's syndrome

- Active alcoholism
  —May show many clinical or biochemical features of Cushing's syndrome, with raised UFC, loss of circadian rhythm and reduced dexamethasone suppressibility, but normal cortisol response to IST
  —biochemistry normalizes rapidly after alcohol withdrawal
- Severe depression
  —Not usually clinically cushingoid, but same biochemistry as alcoholism and normal cortisol response to IST
  —Biochemistry normalizes with antidepressant therapy, unlike Cushing's syndrome

Cyclical Cushing's syndrome

- Between 5 and 10% of all causes of Cushing's syndrome
  —All biochemistry may be normal
  —Repeat UFC at least weekly over several months
- Disparity between clinical and biochemical features

---

recovers by about 2 years following successful surgery in the absence of other hormone deficiencies. It should also be remembered that there is a significant recurrence rate (variably reported as 5–10%), even following seemingly successful surgery, so long-term follow-up is necessary.

Bilateral adrenalectomy and pituitary radiotherapy

If pituitary surgery is unsuccessful or contraindicated, consideration may be given to bilateral adrenalectomy, which, although curative, will require that the individual receives lifelong glucocorticoid and mineralocorticoid replacement. Pituitary irradiation will also be required to reduce the risk of developing Nelson's syndrome (gross hyperpigmentation with very high ACTH levels and a progressive increase in size of the residual adenoma, with the associated risk of mass effect problems). Radiotherapy should also be considered when removal of ACTH macroadenomas is incomplete (such lesions tend to be the most aggressive type of pituitary adenoma). Of course, the risks of pituitary irradiation remain as described previously.

Medical therapy

As yet, there is no consistently effective, long-term medical treatment for Cushing's disease. When severe, temporary medical treatment should be considered prior to definitive therapy in order to improve the patient's overall condition. Most commonly, metyrapone (11-β-hydroxylase inhibitor) can be used in this situation (up to 375 mg q.i.d.), but nausea is not uncommon (reduced by taking with food) and the development of resistance can be a problem. Dose titration should be undertaken to normalize daily urinary free cortisol levels. Some centres use a block replacement regimen with metyrapone and replacement doses of glucocorticoids (dexamethasone preferably, because there is no interference in the cortisol assay). Ketoconazole is an imidazole antifungal drug that is also a potent inhibitor of adrenal steroidogenesis. It can be used alone (building up to 200–400 mg t.d.s.) or in combination with metyrapone (lower doses of each drug may be required), and careful monitoring for the development of hypoadrenalism and/or liver function abnormalities is required.

The more toxic adrenolytic drug mitotane (o,p'-DDD), which both inhibits 11-β-hydroxylase and is toxic to adrenal cortical cells, is usually reserved for the treatment of patients with inoperable malignant ectopic ACTH syndrome or metastatic adrenal carcinoma.

GONADOTROPHIN- AND TSH-SECRETING PITUITARY ADENOMAS

Most so-called NFPAs contain and/or secrete small amounts of both LH and FSH. Although described by some as gonadotrophinomas, this term can be misleading because they do not produce any clinical hormone excess syndrome. True FSH or LH hypersecretion by pituitary adenomas, sufficient to cause a clinical syndrome, is exceptionally rare. When this does occur, children may develop precocious puberty, while men may develop increased testicular size (FSH) or increased testosterone and changes in libido (LH). In premenopausal women, FSH-secreting adenomas may cause ovarian hyperstimulation with increased oestradiol levels.

Likewise, TSH-secreting pituitary adenomas causing hyperthyroidism are exceptionally rare, accounting for no more than 3% of all pituitary adenomas. Patients have often been misdiagnosed previously as having Graves' disease due to the smooth goitre with elevated thyroid hormone levels. However, in primary hyperthyroidism TSH levels are low or undetectable, whereas TSH-secreting adenomas must always be excluded when thyroid hormone levels are elevated in the face of normal or raised TSH levels. A further important distinction is between a true TSH-secreting adenoma and thyroid hormone resistance (pituitary or generalized) due to a range of thyroid hormone receptor mutations. In most patients (90%) with TSH-secreting adenomas:

- the α subunit:intact TSH molar ratio is greater than 1 (excluding those with primary hypogonadism and elevated LH/FSH levels who also have raised α subunit levels)
- the TSH response to TRH is reduced
- sex hormone-binding globulin levels are elevated
- there is radiological evidence of a pituitary adenoma.

When a pituitary adenoma is identified, trans-sphenoidal surgery is the treatment of choice, but alternative and/or additional approaches to the treatment of TSH-secreting adenomas include DA agonists (occasional patients respond) or somatostatin analogue therapy (up to 60% may show some degree of response).

Further reading

Casanueva FP et al. 2006 Guidelines of the Pituitary Society for the diagnosis and management of prolactinomas. Clin Endocrinol 65: 265–273

Ho K, Chihara K (eds) 2006 Molecular pathogenesis and therapy of pituitary disease. Bioscientifica, Bristol.

National Institute for Health and Clinical Excellence 2003 TA64: growth hormone deficiency (adults) – human growth hormone: guidance. NICE, London

Newell-Price J, Bertagna X, Grossman AB et al. 2006 Cushing's syndrome. Lancet 367: 1605–1617

Newell-Price J, Trainer P, Besser M et al. 1998 The diagnosis and differential diagnosis of Cushing's syndrome and pseudo-Cushing's states. Endocr Rev 19: 647–672

Royal College of Physicians 1997 Pituitary tumours: recommendations for service provision and guidelines for management of patients. Consensus of a working party. RCP, London

Wierman ME (ed.) 1997 Diseases of the pituitary: diagnosis and treatment. Humana, New Jersey

SELF-ASSESSMENT

Patient 1

A 46-year-old man is referred because of headaches and enlargement of his hands and feet. He is otherwise perfectly well, but on examination he is mildly acromegalic, confirmed by GH values of 20 mU/L that do not suppress during a glucose tolerance test, together with a raised IGF-1 level (90 mmol/L). His carbohydrate tolerance is normal and he is normotensive. Pituitary MRI showed a 9 mm intrasellar adenoma.

Questions
1. What further information do you need?
2. How would you treat this patient?

Answers
1. The diagnosis of mild acromegaly is confirmed by the glucose tolerance test findings and raised IGF-1 level, but it is important also to know the PRL level. In this case, the PRL was markedly elevated, at 6000 mU/L, and the patient also had hypogonadotrophic hypogonadism but was biochemically euthyroid.
2. This level of PRL is too high for stalk compression hyperprolactinaemia and, in any event, microadenomas do not cause stalk compression. It is most likely that the patient has a PRL/GH-secreting mammosomatotroph adenoma. The treatment of choice is not trans-sphenoidal surgery but a trial of DA agonist therapy.

The patient was commenced on cabergoline (0.5 mg twice weekly); his headaches disappeared, and repeat assessment at 3 months showed normalization of GH, IGF-1 and PRL, normal gonadal function and disappearance of the microadenoma on repeat MRI.

Although DA agonist therapy is not relevant for most patients with acromegaly, it is important not to miss those with significant hyperprolactinaemia who may respond well to this treatment.

Patient 2

A 35-year-old woman is referred with 3 months' secondary amenorrhoea and galactorrhoea. She is tired, with headache and hot flushes. Investigation at her local hospital revealed hyperprolactinaemia (3500 mU/L), a negative pregnancy test, hypogonadotrophic hypogonadism and pituitary enlargement with a small suprasellar extension on MRI, as shown in Figure 1.7.

Questions
1. What further information do you require?
2. How would you treat her?

Figure 1.7
Pituitary CT prior to treatment.

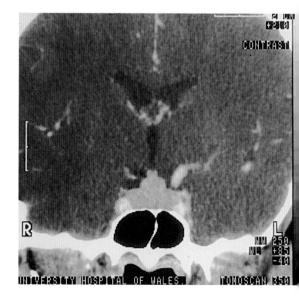

Figure 1.8
Pituitary CT 3 months after commencing thyroxine replacement.

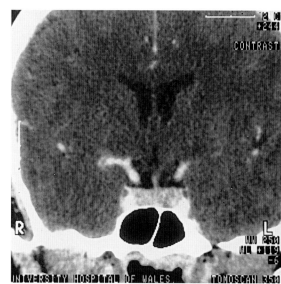

Answer

It would be a great mistake to commence this patient on any DA agonist treatment at this stage. The crucial missing piece of information is the result of thyroid function testing. Her free T_4 was 4 pmol/L, with a basal TSH greater than 50 mU/L. Although she presented with galactorrhoea and amenorrhoea, she did give a history commensurate with long-standing hypothyroidism, but this was not elicited initially. People were sidetracked by the neuroradiology findings and misled into thinking that this was a prolactinoma. After treatment with T_4 for 3 months, repeat radiology showed a normal pituitary gland (Fig. 1.8). The initial pituitary enlargement was purely the result of long-standing thyrotroph hyperplasia.

Disorders of growth, puberty and sexual differentiation

2

J. H. Davies and J. W. Gregory

LINEAR GROWTH

Physiology of normal growth

Fetal growth is critical in determining the final height of an individual. In utero, the growth of the fetus is mediated by factors such as insulin, insulin-like growth factor (IGF)-1 and IGF-2 and also maternal nutrition, and growth at this time is largely independent of endogenous growth hormone (GH) secretion. Compromised production of these factors or maternal nutrition is associated with intrauterine growth retardation. However, during infancy nutritional status is the predominant influence on linear growth. Thereafter, the GH–IGF-1 axis becomes the major endocrine regulator of linear growth.

Normal linear growth

Postnatal linear growth can be divided into three phases: infancy, childhood and puberty. Throughout infancy, linear growth is rapid, although height velocity decreases markedly (Fig. 2.1). Furthermore, during the first 2 years a period of catch-up or catch-down growth commonly takes place as the individuals establish their own growth trajectory. The childhood growth pattern extends from preschool until the onset of puberty. During this time, hormonal influences on growth predominate, particularly the GH–IGF-1 axis. Normal height velocity in mid-childhood ranges from 4 to 8 cm/year, with little sexual dimorphism in growth until the onset of puberty.

The pubertal growth spurt occurs as a result of increasing sex steroid production from hypothalamopituitary–gonadal activation and also from a further increase in GH secretion. In girls, the growth spurt starts approximately 2 years earlier than in boys, and the onset coincides with the start of breast development. In females, peak height velocity (8 cm/year) occurs around 12 years of age and is followed by the onset of menarche, after which height velocity decelerates, with approximately 2 years' growth (around 5 cm) left till the attainment of final height.

By contrast, in boys the onset of the pubertal growth spurt occurs well into puberty, when testicular volumes are 10–12 mL. Peak height velocity (10 cm/year) occurs around

Figure 2.1
Height velocity during infancy, childhood and puberty.

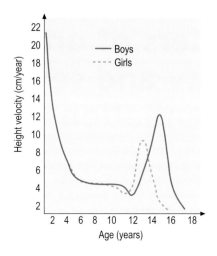

Figure 2.2
Non-pathological influences on growth. GH, growth hormone.

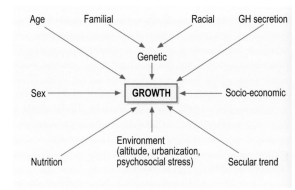

14 years of age, when testicular volumes are 15 mL. When linear growth ceases, testicular volumes are around 20 mL. Males are on average 13–14 cm taller than females as a result of two additional years of prepubertal growth and a greater peak height velocity during puberty.

The final stature of an individual results from the interaction between factors such as genes, environmental factors, the hormonal milieu and nutritional status (Fig. 2.2).

SHORT STATURE

Short stature is arbitrarily defined as a height that lies two standard deviations below the mean (equating to below the second centile) for the child's age and gender, compared with the normal population. Assessment of an individual's genetic background is made by calculation of the target height centile range using parental heights (Box 2.1).

Box 2.1: Clinical evaluation of short stature

History

- Family history of short stature or consanguinity
- Family history of delayed puberty
- Birth weight and gestation
- Neonatal history of jaundice or hypoglycaemia (suggestive of hypopituitarism)
- Systematic enquiry, including:
  —symptoms of gastrointestinal disturbance
  —symptoms of hypothyroidism
- Social history and school performance

Examination

- Height, weight, sitting height to be plotted on centile chart; calculation of decimal age and height velocity
- Heights of parents to calculate target centile range:

$$[\text{mother's height (cm)} + \text{father's height (cm)}]/2 = \sigma$$

—For boys:

$$\text{mid-parental height} = \sigma + 7\ \text{cm} = \lambda$$

$$\text{target centile range} = \lambda \pm 10\ \text{cm}$$

—For girls:

$$\text{mid-parental height} = \sigma - 7\ \text{cm} = \gamma$$

$$\text{target centile range} = \gamma \pm 10\ \text{cm}$$

- Pubertal status
- Signs of dysmorphism

Clinical evaluation and investigation of short stature

The majority of children with short stature do not have an underlying hormonal or genetic abnormality and do not require further investigation (Box 2.2). There are certain clinical features, however, that may suggest the need for further investigation (Box 2.3). A thorough history and examination should be taken, seeking symptoms suggestive of chronic disease and associated features of chromosomal disorders or other syndromes. The clinical assessment will determine subsequent investigations (Boxes 2.1 and 2.4). The importance of undertaking accurate auxology cannot be overemphasized, and the reader is referred to standard growth charts for further instruction. A persistent reduction in height velocity over 1 year (therefore taking into account seasonal variation of growth) can be a sensitive indicator of disease (see *Further reading, Overview of paediatric endocrinology*).

Measurement of length and height

Measuring equipment should be regularly calibrated and checked for accuracy prior to each clinic session. The measurer should be trained in standard auxological techniques, and ideally the same individual should make the measurements each time to minimize errors. For babies and infants under 2 years of age, a supine measurement is undertaken and two people are needed to make an accurate measurement. From the age of 2 years, a stadiometer is used to measure linear growth. The subject stands with heels (without

Box 2.2: Causes of short stature

- Familial short stature
- Constitutional delay of growth and puberty
- Short stature following intrauterine growth retardation
- Chronic disease:
  —inflammatory bowel disease
  —coeliac disease
  —chronic renal failure
- Psychosocial deprivation
- Dysmorphic syndromes:
  —Turner's syndrome
  —Russell–Silver syndrome
  —Noonan syndrome
  —Prader–Willi syndrome
  —pseudohypoparathyroidism type 1a
- Skeletal dysplasia
- Endocrine disorders:
  —growth hormone deficiency
  —hypothyroidism
  —Cushing's syndrome
  —growth hormone resistance

Box 2.3: Clinical features suggesting the need for further investigation in short stature

- Extreme short stature
- Height significantly below the target height (>1.4 SD below mid-parental height)
- Subnormal height velocity (height velocity SD score <0 over 1 year)
- History of symptoms suggesting chronic disease
- Dysmorphic features
- Precocious or delayed puberty

Box 2.4: Investigation of short stature

Baseline tests

- Full blood count
- Erythrocyte sedimentation rate/C-reactive protein
- Urea, creatinine, electrolytes
- Calcium, phosphate, liver function tests
- Ferritin, serum immunoglobulin A, anti-tissue transglutaminase antibodies
- Karyotype (girls)
- Thyroid function test
- Insulin-like growth factor (IGF)-1, IGF binding protein-3
- Prolactin
- Skeletal survey in dysmorphic children
- Bone age x-ray

If baseline investigations are normal *and* height velocity subnormal, consider growth hormone dynamic testing.

shoes or socks), buttocks and shoulder blades against the back plate, and the measurer ensures that the imaginary line from the centre of the external auditory meatus to the lower border of the eye socket (the Frankfurt plane) is horizontal. The measurer then applies pressure on the mastoid processes, and the reading is taken at maximum extension without the heels losing contact with the baseboard. The height should be plotted on a growth chart using a decimal age.

Familial short stature

The commonest cause of short stature is familial, the diagnosis usually being made on the basis of:

- a height standard deviation score that lies within the target centile range calculated from parental heights
- the exclusion of disease based on clinical and biochemical parameters.

Mutations of the SHOX gene and the GHR gene have been identified in some individuals with familial short stature.

Constitutional delay of growth and puberty

See p. 48.

Dysmorphic syndromes

Turner's syndrome

Turner's syndrome is a disorder in females characterized by the absence of all or part of a normal second sex chromosome, which leads to a constellation of physical findings that include short stature and gonadal dysgenesis. It occurs in one in 2500 live-born girls. The final height in these individuals may be increased by human GH administration (Table 2.1). Sex hormone replacement is usually required for completion of puberty.

Prader–Willi syndrome

Children with Prader–Willi syndrome have hypothalamic dysregulation, which results in abnormalities in satiety, growth, energy expenditure and sleep. Exogenous human GH administration may be used for improving growth and body composition (Table 2.1).

Table 2.1: Recommended doses for growth hormone therapy in children

Indication	Dose (mg/kg per day)
Growth hormone deficiency	0.025–0.035
Chronic renal insufficiency	0.045–0.050
Turner's syndrome	0.045–0.050
Prader–Willi syndrome	0.035
Small for gestational age	0.035

Treatment is discontinued when height velocity is <2 cm/year or at final height.

Russell–Silver syndrome

This disorder is a cause of intrauterine growth retardation. Dysmorphic features include a prominent forehead and triangular face, and asymmetry of the limbs. Maternal parental disomy of chromosome 7 is thought to be causal in approximately 10% of patients with Russell–Silver syndrome.

Endocrine disorders

Growth hormone deficiency

Growth hormone deficiency is the commonest endocrine disorder that presents with short stature, and occurs in one in 4000 people. There are many known causes of growth hormone deficiency, but most cases are idiopathic (Box 2.5). The clinical features of childhood-onset growth hormone deficiency are:

• subnormal height velocity
• excess subcutaneous fat
• mid-facial hypoplasia
• delayed skeletal maturation.

Associated features include micropenis, hypoglycaemia and symptoms of wider pituitary dysfunction. Treatment is with human GH (Table 2.1).

Other endocrine disorders

There are many other endocrine disorders that can lead to short stature, including acquired hypothyroidism. Linear growth may be suppressed by elevated cortisol concentrations in Cushing's syndrome. More rarely, GH resistance (Laron syndrome, a growth hormone receptor mutation) leads to extreme short stature.

Box 2.5: Causes of growth hormone deficiency

Acquired

• Central nervous system tumours: craniopharyngioma, germinoma, optic glioma
• Histiocytosis
• Cranial irradiation
• Head injury
• Inflammatory/granulomatous diseases

Genetic

• Growth hormone-1 mutations
• Growth hormone-releasing hormone receptor mutations
• PIT-1, POUF-1 mutations

Transient

• Psychosocial deprivation
• Hypothyroidism
• Prepubertal

PUBERTY

Physiology of normal puberty

Puberty is the physical transition from childhood to adulthood that results in reproductive capability. Normally, it occurs between the ages of 8 and 13 years in girls and 9 and 14 years in boys. The majority of the variation in pubertal timing cannot be attributed to any clinical disorder (Fig. 2.3), even after extensive investigation. Mutations of genes have been identified that provide insight into the underlying physiology (Box 2.6).

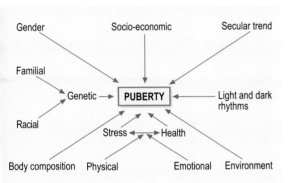

Figure 2.3
Non-pathological influences on pubertal timing.

Box 2.6: Monogenic disorders of puberty

Genetic defects causing precocious puberty

- Luteinizing hormone receptor-activating mutations
- 21-Hydroxylase, 11-hydroxylase and 3-β-hydroxysteroid dehydrogenase mutations
- Aromatase gene promoter aberrant function
- Glucocorticoid receptor gene mutations
- Gs α subunit-activating somatic mutations (McCune–Albright syndrome)

Gene mutations that cause delayed puberty

- KAL-1
- DAX-1
- GPR-54
- SF-1
- PC-1
- PROP-1
- FSH-β
- FSHR
- LH-β
- LHR
- Oestrogen receptor
- Androgen receptor
- 5-α-Reductase
- Aromatase
- 17-Hydroxylase, 17,20-desmolase, 20,22-desmolase, StAR
- HSD17B3

The onset of puberty is controlled by several neuroendocrine factors and hormones that regulate the hypothalamic gonadotrophin-releasing hormone (GnRH) pulse generator. GnRH stimulates the release of follicle-stimulating hormone (FSH) and luteinizing hormone (LH) from the gonadotrophs of the anterior pituitary into the systemic circulation. The resultant physical changes of puberty result from sex steroid action on the body (Fig. 2.4 and Table 2.2). In both sexes during this time, increased sex steroid and insulin production enhance the secretion of GH and IGF-1.

Girls

FSH stimulates follicle formation and oestrogen production, whereas LH stimulates progesterone secretion after the onset of ovulation. Puberty begins with breast enlargement at a mean age of 11 years. This is followed by pubic and axillary hair development and then menarche, the latter of these occurring at a mean age of 13.5 years. The pubertal growth spurt starts early in pubertal development, at breast stage 2–3, and usually within the first year of pubertal onset.

Boys

LH stimulates Leydig cell secretion of testosterone, and FSH stimulates spermatogenesis by the Sertoli cells. Inhibin B, produced by Sertoli cells, exerts a negative feedback on FSH secretion. Sex hormone-binding globulin concentrations fall so that free androgen concentrations rise. Puberty begins with testicular enlargement (attainment of 4 mL of testicular volume), normally between the ages of 9 and 14 years and at a mean age of 12 years. This is followed by pubic and axillary hair development. The average time between first pubertal signs and mature development is 3 years. The pubertal growth spurt occurs later in pubertal development compared with in girls, at a testicular volume of around 12 mL.

Terminology

- *Gonadarche:* the activation of gonads that results in secretion of sex hormones.
- *Oligomenorrhoea:* infrequent periods (fewer than six per year).
- *Menarche:* the onset of periods.
- *Pubarche:* the appearance of pubic hair.
- *Thelarche:* the onset of breast development.

Precocious puberty

Precocious puberty is defined as the onset of puberty before the age of 8 years in girls and 9 years in boys. Gonadotrophin-dependent precocious puberty (GDPP) is the development of secondary sexual characteristics in the normal sequence resulting from activation of the hypothalamus but occurring abnormally early. By contrast, gonadotrophin-independent precocious puberty (GIPP) is the result of abnormal production of sex steroids, which is independent of hypothalamic–pituitary activation. GIPP may result in non-consonant puberty, i.e. puberty occurring in an abnormal sequence (Box 2.7).

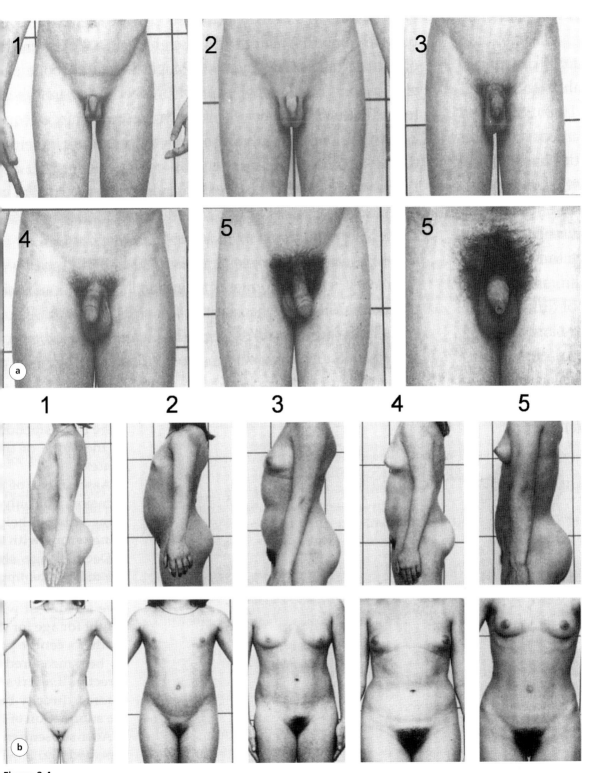

Figure 2.4
Stages of **(a)** male and **(b)** female puberty. From Brook, Clayton, Brown, Brook's Clinical Pediatric Endocrinology, 5e, with permission from Blackwell Publishing.

Table 2.2: Stages of puberty

Stage	Definition
Breast staging	
B1	Prepubertal
B2	Breast budding, small amount of glandular tissue, areola widens
B3	Development of actual breast mound, areola continues to enlarge but remains in contour with the breast
B4	Areola and papilla project at an angle to breast mound
B5	Adult configuration, areola and breast in same plane with papilla projecting above the areola
Genital staging	
G1	Prepubertal penis (unstretched length 2.5–6 cm), testes volume ≤3 mL
G2	Testes ≥4 mL ± scrotal laxity but no penile enlargement
G3	Penile lengthening, with further development of the testes and scrotum
G4	Penile lengthening and broadening, darkening of scrotum, testes usually 10–12 mL
G5	Adult genitalia, testes 15–25 mL
Pubic hair staging	
PH1	No pubic hair
PH2	Fine hair over mons and/or labia/scrotum
PH3	Adult-type hair but distribution confined to pubis
PH4	Extension to near-adult distribution
PH5	Adult distribution
Axillary hair staging	
A1	No axillary hair
A2	Hair present but not adult content
A3	Adult content

Clinical evaluation and investigation of precocious puberty

The clinical assessment of precocious puberty should distinguish whether the symptoms and signs are related to excess secretion of androgens, oestrogens or both, and establish an underlying cause when possible. Enquiry about specific symptomatology related to causal factors should be sought, and a detailed examination with auxology should be undertaken (Box 2.8). The history and clinical evaluation will determine the subsequent investigations (Box 2.9). The luteinizing hormone-releasing hormone (LHRH) test is particularly helpful in distinguishing GDPP from GIPP, as basal gonadotrophins may be low in both.

Gonadotrophin-dependent precocious puberty

In general, GDPP is more common in girls than in boys. In girls, 95% of cases of GDPP are idiopathic, whereas in boys GDPP is much more likely to have a pathological cause. Pathological causes of GDPP occur more frequently in those presenting before 5 years of age and with rapid pubertal progression (Box 2.7).

Box 2.7: Causes of precocious puberty

Gonadotrophin-dependent puberty

- Idiopathic
- Secondary:
  —cerebral palsy/hydrocephalus
  —hypothalamic tumour
  —head trauma
  —cranial irradiation
  —sexual abuse
  —adoption-related

Gonadotrophin-independent puberty

Precocious breast development

- Premature thelarche
- Thelarche variant
- Hypothyroidism

Virilization (pubic/axillary hair development)

- Adrenarche
- Congenital adrenal hyperplasia
- Cushing's disease
- Adrenal tumours

Others

- Premature menarche
- Gonadotrophin-secreting tumours/sex steroid-secreting tumours
- McCune–Albright syndrome
- Testoxicosis
- Pubic hair of infancy
- Exogenous steroids

Box 2.8: Clinical evaluation of precocious puberty

History

- Androgen-mediated symptoms/signs: greasy hair, body odour, acne, pubic/axillary hair, enlargement of penis/clitoris, accelerated linear growth, mood swings
- Oestrogen-mediated symptoms/signs: breast development, vaginal bleeding and discharge, accelerated linear growth, mood swings
- Secondary causes: headache, vomiting, visual disturbance, previous neurosurgery, cranial irradiation, history of hydrocephalus, cerebral palsy

Examination

- Height standard deviation score and weight standard deviation score
- Pubertal status
- Blood pressure
- Neurological examination including fundoscopy
- Visual fields
- Neurocutaneous stigmata

Box 2.9: Investigation of precocious puberty

Initial investigations of girls with breast development[a] or boys with testicular enlargement[b]

- Luteinizing hormone-releasing hormone test (only if basal gonadotrophins not diagnostically elevated)
- Oestradiol (girls), testosterone (boys)
- Thyroid function test
- In girls, pelvic ultrasound for uterine and ovarian dimensions and evidence of endometrial stripe and ovarian follicles
- Consider:
  —bone age
  —magnetic resonance imaging (MRI) of head if GDPP

If clinical assessment and initial investigations suggest oestrogen-mediated GIPP

- β-Human chorionic gonadotrophin (β-hCG)
- α-Fetoprotein
- Urine for steroid metabolites (feminizing adrenal tumour)

If clinical assessment and initial investigations suggest androgen-mediated GIPP

- Testosterone
- 17-Hydroxyprogesterone
- Androstenedione
- Dehydroepiandrosterone
- Urine for steroid metabolites
- Consider:
  —standard synacthen test with measurement of basal and stimulated adrenal androgens
  —β-hCG and α-fetoprotein
  —adrenal computerized tomography and MRI
  —dexamethasone suppression test

GDPP, gonadotrophin-dependent precocious puberty; GIPP, gonadotrophin-independent precocious puberty.
[a]That is, potentially GDPP or GIPP.
[b]Usually indicating GDPP.

Management of gonadotrophin-dependent precocious puberty

Treatment is with a GnRH analogue until 11 years of age. GnRH analogues occupy the GnRH receptor and prevent pulsatile gonadotrophin secretion. Treatment prevents pubertal progression and indirectly prevents premature epiphyseal closure, thus allowing continued linear growth. The indications for treatment include poor final height prognosis and prevention of perceived psychological distress to the individual of pubertal progression at a young age. Regular follow-up is required, including auxology, annual bone age and in girls a pelvic ultrasound.

Gonadotrophin-independent precocious puberty

Gonadotrophin-independent precocious puberty is rare, and pathological causes must be excluded (Box 2.7). In girls, differentiating GDPP from GIPP by clinical evaluation is difficult, as both may present initially with breast development. Rarely, human chorionic gonadotrophin-secreting tumours in boys also give the clinical picture of GDPP, but the LHRH test will demonstrate GIPP. There are certain clinical entities that are considered a variant of normal puberty and that usually do not require treatment, and these are discussed below.

Premature thelarche

Premature thelarche is the appearance of breast tissue (B2) in a girl under 3 years of age with normal growth and without evidence of rapid pubertal progression over time and no evidence of a central nervous system problem. There may be an exaggerated FSH response to an LHRH test, but all other investigations will be normal and no treatment is required.

Thelarche variant

Thelarche variant is a descriptive term for girls in whom thelarche is persistent or slowly progressive, often associated with a moderate increase in height velocity and bone age and sometimes vaginal bleeding, but with a prepubertal response to an LHRH test. Regular follow-up is necessary to evaluate the rapidity of pubertal progression. For more severe cases, cyproterone acetate treatment may be considered but is often ineffective.

Premature menarche

Premature menarche is the occurrence of one or more episodes of vaginal bleeding in a girl aged 4–8 years with no breast development and no abnormal physical findings, hormonal studies or imaging findings. Other causes of vaginal bleeding must be excluded (e.g. foreign body, vulvovaginitis, sexual abuse or tumour).

Premature adrenarche

Premature adrenarche is defined as the appearance of pubic and/or axillary hair in the absence of thelarche or testicular development, associated with adrenal androgen production, before the age of 8 years in girls and 9 years in boys. The majority have a normal growth rate, although rapid growth may be noted initially. It is the commonest cause of isolated pubic hair development in girls and boys. As no treatment is required for adrenarche, it is important to distinguish it from 21-hydroxylase deficiency. During childhood, premature adrenarche is associated with reduced insulin sensitivity in both sexes. Furthermore, girls with premature adrenarche have an increased predisposition to polycystic ovary disease.

Other causes of gonadotrophin-independent precocious puberty

Congenital adrenal hyperplasia due to 21-hydroxylase deficiency is the commonest pathological cause of androgen-mediated sexual precocity. Rapid pubertal progression in the presence of a prepubertal LHRH test suggests the presence of a malignancy such as an adrenal adenoma or ovarian granulosa cell tumour, which will require surgical removal. GIPP with multiple café au lait pigmentation indicates McCune–Albright syndrome.

Management of gonadotrophin-independent precocious puberty

Medical management of these patients is often challenging, and continued surveillance is necessary to evaluate the response to treatment. Medical treatment of GIPP is directed at restricting or antagonizing sex steroid production with agents such as cyproterone acetate, testolactone and/or aromatase inhibitors. Delayed treatment of GIPP may be associated with activation of the hypothalamopituitary–gonadal axis and development of GDPP, which may also require treatment with a GnRH analogue.

Delayed puberty

Delayed puberty is defined as the absence of secondary sexual characteristics by 13 years in girls or 14 years in boys, or primary amenorrhoea by age 15 years in girls. Delayed puberty has many causes and is more likely to be pathological in girls than in boys. The causes can be subdivided into those with inappropriately low gonadotrophins (hypogonadotrophic hypogonadism) or those with inappropriately high gonadotrophins (hypergonadotrophic hypogonadism) (Box 2.10).

Clinical evaluation and investigation of delayed puberty

The aim of the clinical assessment of delayed puberty is to evaluate whether delayed puberty or lack of pubertal progression is a result of a normal lag in pubertal maturation or an abnormality that requires further investigation (Boxes 2.11 and 2.12). The majority of individuals presenting with delayed puberty do not require further investigation.

Hypogonadotrophic hypogonadism

Constitutional delay of growth and puberty

This is a variant of normal and is more common in boys than in girls. This may be because constitutional delay of growth and puberty (CDGP) is associated with short stature, which may result in greater psychological morbidity in boys. There is often a family history of delayed puberty, and the bone age is delayed. The biochemical investigations confirm hypogonadotrophic hypogonadism but no other abnormalities.

Hypergonadotrophic hypogonadism

Chromosomal abnormalities

Turner's syndrome is the commonest cause of primary gonadal failure in girls. Some of these girls will spontaneously enter puberty, but few will complete it. Boys with Klinefelter syndrome are often tall and may have a history of behavioural disturbance. Pubertal onset is often spontaneous, but full virilization is not completed and it is unusual for testicular volumes to exceed 8–10 mL. In both disorders, infertility is usual.

Acquired gonadal failure

The commonest cause is prior radiotherapy or chemotherapy administration. Rarely, autoimmunity may cause gonadal failure.

Management of hypogonadism

Treatment of CDGP is instituted if the wider impact of delayed pubertal development, in terms of psychological well-being, is likely to have an adverse effect on the individual. It

Box 2.10: Causes of delayed puberty

Hypogonadotrophic hypogonadism

- Constitutional delay of growth and puberty
- Congenital
- Central nervous system defects (e.g. septo-optic dysplasia)
- Kallmann's syndrome
- DAX-1 mutations

Acquired

- Hypothalamic/pituitary tumours
- Radiotherapy
- Surgery
- Trauma

Syndromic

- Noonan syndrome
- Prader–Willi syndrome

Others

- Anorexia
- Inflammatory bowel disease
- Cystic fibrosis
- Chronic renal failure

Hypergonadotrophic hypogonadism

Chromosomal abnormalities

- Turner's syndrome (45, XO)
- Klinefelter syndrome (47, XXY)

Disorders of gonadal/sexual development

- Pure and partial gonadal dysgenesis
- Mixed gonadal dysgenesis (45, XO/46, XX)
- Steroid biosynthetic defects
- Gonadal agenesis

Acquired gonadal failure

- Gonadal radiotherapy
- Chemotherapy
- Torsion
- Postmumps orchitis
- Previous orchidopexy
- Autoimmune

Others

- Galactosaemia
- Mucopolysaccharidosis
- Luteinizing hormone/follicle-stimulating hormone resistance

is also important to engage in a discussion with the patient and family regarding realistic treatment expectations (Box 2.13). Treatment is with testosterone in boys and oestrogen in girls at low dose for 4–12 months, after which pubertal progression should become evident. Treatment of CDGP does not compromise final height.

Box 2.11: Clinical evaluation of delayed puberty

History

- Signs or symptoms of chronic disease
- Family history of delayed puberty
- Headache
- Visual disturbance
- Symptoms of hypothyroidism

Examination

- Presence of dysmorphism
- Height standard deviation score and weight standard deviation score
- Pubertal status
- Visual fields
- Neurological examination including fundoscopy
- Skeletal disproportion

Box 2.12: Investigation of delayed puberty

- Full blood count, C-reactive protein, erythrocyte sedimentation rate
- Urea and electrolytes, creatinine
- LH, FSH, testosterone
- Prolactin
- Thyroid function tests
- Karyotype
- Consider:
  —bone age
  —ultrasound study of pelvis (females)
  —luteinizing hormone-releasing hormone test

Box 2.13: Indications for medical treatment of constitutional delay of growth and puberty

- Short stature
- Low height velocity
- Delayed secondary sexual development
- Abnormal body proportions
- Reduced bone mineral density
- Psychological disturbance:
  —poor self-image
  —looking and feeling different to peers
  —lack of confidence
  —depression
  —school refusal
  —aggressiveness and delinquency
  —reduced employment opportunities
- Parental concern

For persistent causes of hypogonadism, treatment is with an increasing dose of sex steroids over 2–3 years to full adult replacement doses to complete pubertal development. Regular clinical evaluation is essential to monitor the progression of puberty, as prolongation of insufficient dosing leads to further pubertal delay and excessive dosing or rapid increases may lead to inadequate breast and uterine development in girls. Hormone replacement is then continued into adulthood.

SEXUAL DETERMINATION AND DIFFERENTIATION

Physiology of sexual differentiation

In males and females, the indifferent gonad develops from the genital ridge (Fig. 2.5). Migrating primordial germ cells reach the ridge by 6–8 weeks' gestation. Genetic sex is determined at conception and controls the differentiation of the gonad. Testicular differentiation and testosterone production occur by 9 weeks' gestation, whereas ovarian differentiation and germ cell meiosis occur by 11–12 weeks' gestation. Sex differentiation involves the development of the internal genitalia, the urogenital sinus and external genitalia, partly under endocrine regulation (Fig. 2.5).

Female differentiation of the fetus will occur unless there is expression of specific genes and hormones that control testicular differentiation and the subsequent development of male internal and external genitalia. Furthermore, the gonads may exert a paracrine effect on adjacent tissues; testes, for example, cause wolffian duct development and regression of müllerian structures. An important point is that the presence of a uterus in a newborn with ambiguous genitalia indicates that an ovary or a dysgenetic testis is present, or there is no gonad.

Terminology

- *Sex determination:* the formation of a gonad as a testis or an ovary.
- *Sex differentiation:* the development of physical characteristics, both internal and external, as a result of gonad function.
- *Ambiguous genitalia:* a form of intersex in which the sexual phenotype does not allow the clinical assignment of gender.
- *Hermaphroditism:* the presence in one individual of both testicular (with seminiferous tubules) and ovarian tissue (with follicles), which may be in separate gonads or ovotestes.
- *Gender assignment:* 'becoming' male or female at birth.
- *Gender identity:* the sense of self as male or female.
- *Gender role:* aspects of behaviour attributed to males or females.
- *Sexual orientation:* the target of sexual arousal.
- *Gender dysphoria:* a transsexual state.

Recently, there has been a change to the nomenclature of the various descriptions of genital anomalies. The change was proposed as a result of terms such as

51

Figure 2.5
(a) Male and **(b)** female development.

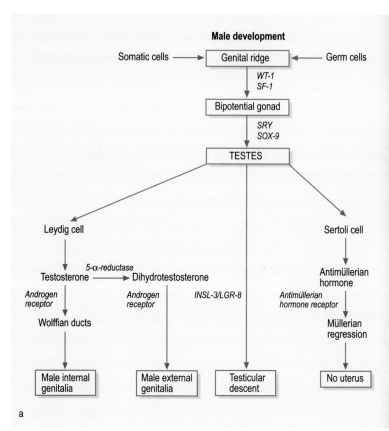

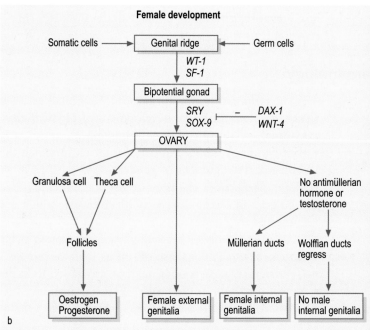

pseudohermaphroditism leading to diagnostic confusion and also affected individuals stating that such terminology was unacceptable to them. The term *disorders of sex development* (DSD) is now used and is defined as congenital conditions in which development of chromosomal, gonadal or anatomical sex is atypical. For a more detailed description of the new nomenclature, the reader is referred to the consensus statement on the management of intersex disorders (see *Further reading*).

Aetiology of disorders of sex development

The causes of disorders of sexual differentiation can be classified clinically as masculinized females, undermasculinized males and true hermaphroditism (Table 2.3). The commonest cause of ambiguous genitalia at birth is 21-hydroxylase deficiency, which results in a masculinized female phenotype. However, in the majority of cases of XY intersex no cause is identified. Even though genital anomalies occur in one in 4500 births, the presentation of intersex is not confined to the newborn period. Non-isosexual development can occur at puberty with 17-β-hydroxysteroid dehydrogenase deficiency, 5-α-reductase deficiency, late-onset congenital adrenal hyperplasia and partial androgen insensitivity.

Table 2.3: Clinical classification and aetiology of intersex disorders

Phenotype	Aetiology
Masculinized XX female (46, XX DSD)	21-Hydroxylase deficiency
	11-β-Hydroxylase deficiency
	3-β-Hydroxysteroid dehydrogenase deficiency
	Placental aromatase deficiency
	Adrenal tumours
	Ovarian tumours
Undermasculinized XY male (46, XY DSD)	
Failure in gonad determination	Gonadal dysgenesis
	XO/XY mosaicism
Failure in androgen biosynthesis	StAR protein deficiency
	3-β-Hydroxysteroid dehydrogenase deficiency
	17-α-Hydroxylase deficiency
	17,20-Desmolase deficiency
	17-β-Hydroxysteroid dehydrogenase deficiency
	Leydig cell hypoplasia (luteinizing hormone deficiency or luteinizing hormone receptor defect)
	Secondary to hypopituitarism
Failure in androgen action	Complete androgen insensitivity syndrome
	Partial androgen insensitivity syndrome
	5-α-Reductase deficiency
True hermaphroditism (ovotesticular DSD)	XX
	XY
	XX/XY

Clinical evaluation and investigation of disorders of sex development

A thorough history and examination should be undertaken, which may give insight into the aetiology of the genital anomaly (Box 2.14). It is not possible to assign gender on the basis of clinical evaluation alone, and biochemical investigations in these individuals are usually required. There are various clinical presentations that require further investigation (Box 2.14). It is essential that there is a discriminatory approach to the investigation of newborns with ambiguous genitalia that is guided by the history and examination and also the age of the baby (Fig. 2.6 and Box 2.15).

Management of disorders of sex development

The initial management of ambiguous genitalia is complex and is considered a medical emergency. The baby should be monitored for hypoglycaemia and salt wasting in the first few days. The aim is to assign gender as early as possible, which involves consultation of the parents with a paediatric endocrinologist, paediatric urologist and psychologist. The infant is referred to as 'your baby' until gender is assigned, although some parents prefer to use a non-gender-specific name during this time. Surgery is appropriate in the first year of life for masculinized females and hypospadias repair in undermasculinized males. A view is emerging that feminizing surgery for undermasculinized males may be inappropriate in terms of the potential for psychological morbidity and adverse sexual health in adulthood of affected individuals.

Box 2.14: Clinical evaluation of disorders of sex development

History

- Maternal medication during pregnancy
- Maternal virilization during pregnancy
- Consanguinity
- Family history of neonatal deaths (undiagnosed adrenal insufficiency) and ambiguous genitalia

Examination

- Size of clitoris/phallus
- Degree of labial fusion
- Position of urethra/urogenital sinus
- Degree of hypospadias
- Are gonads palpable? (Check inguinal canals)
- Examination of anus
- Signs of hypopituitarism (midline defects, hypoglycaemia, hypocortisolism, prolonged jaundice)
- Features of Turner's syndrome may be seen in mosaicism or partial gonadal dysgenesis

Features determining which newborns to investigate

- Ambiguous genitalia
- Severe hypospadias with or without undescended testes, micropenis, bifid/shawl scrotum
- Male with non-palpable testes
- Female with inguinal herniae
- Isolated clitoromegaly
- Isolated labial fusion
- Syndromal genital anomalies
- Electrolyte abnormalities suggestive of adrenal insufficiency

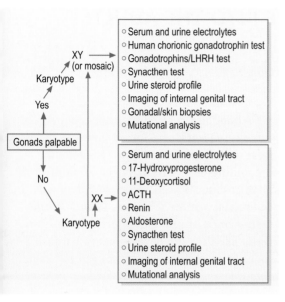

Figure 2.6
Discriminatory approach to the investigation
of disorders of sex development.
ACTH, adrenocorticotrophic hormone;
LHRH, luteinizing hormone-releasing hormone.

Box 2.15: Investigation of ambiguous genitalia

Day 1 of life

- Karyotype
- Daily electrolytes and glucose to monitor for adrenal insufficiency
- Ultrasound study of pelvis to determine presence of müllerian structures and gonads in labial folds

After day 2 of life

- Calculate fractional sodium excretion if adrenal disorder suspected
- 17-Hydroxyprogesterone; consider 11-deoxycorticosterone
- Testosterone, dihydrotestosterone, dehydroepiandrosterone, androstenedione
- Luteinizing hormone and follicle-stimulating hormone
- Thyroid function tests
- Urine for steroid metabolites
- Consider:
  —short synacthen test if masculinized female suspected
  —3-day human chorionic gonadotrophin test if undermasculinized male
  —LHRH test if suspected hypopituitarism (only informative at <6 months of age)
  —clinical photography

At the outset, the family should be informed of the plan for any medical and surgical interventions that may be needed over the coming years. When counselling families regarding gender assignment, it is important to be sensitive to the wider social and cultural implications this may have within different communities. The criteria for consideration of gender assignment include the diagnosis, presence of female structures, adequacy of phallic tissue, potential for fertility, parental wishes and cultural aspects.

TRANSITION OF YOUNG PEOPLE INTO THE ADULT ENDOCRINE SERVICE

Transition can be defined as a purposeful, planned process that addresses the medical, psychosocial and educational needs of adolescents and young adults with chronic physical and medical conditions as they move from child-centred to adult-oriented healthcare systems. For the individual, this time represents a period of physical and social changes that start in late puberty and end with full adult maturation. This roughly equates to starting from mid to late teens and ending 6–7 years after the attainment of final height. Historically, there has been an unmet clinical need for these individuals. In the UK, to address this, the *National Service Framework for Children, Young People and Maternity Services* has highlighted the importance of safe and effective transition throughout children's services and identified the need for the development of transitional services. More recently, guidance for the provision of such services has been published by the Department of Health (see *Further reading*).

During the transition period, young people should be supported to achieve their maximum potential in terms of health, education and well-being. Transition clinics have been shown to be effective in a number of other chronic disease states, including diabetes mellitus, in terms of improving compliance during the handover to adult services and aiding patient acceptance of adult services. Transition care requires a dedicated service with close collaboration between paediatric and adult endocrinologists and other relevant services, including psychology. Evidence is accumulating that such a service will improve continuity of care, enable better disease control, minimize the dropout rate from follow-up, and enable focus on different aspects of care beyond specific endocrine issues. There are various models for transition services that will be governed by local resources.

During consultations at this time, there is greater emphasis placed on the education of young persons about their disease. When appropriate, individuals are encouraged to participate and take responsibility for self-management of their illness. The effect that illness or treatment may have on family planning or career prospects is also discussed. There is already a model for the treatment of young people treated with GH and their transition to adult services (see *Further reading*). However, the principles of transition care should also be applied to all young people who are to be transferred from the paediatric endocrine clinic to the adult endocrine service.

Further reading

Overview of paediatric endocrinology

Brook C, Clayton P, Brown R 2005 Brook's clinical pediatric endocrinology, 5th edn. Blackwell, Oxford
Raine JE, Donaldson MDC, Gregory JW et al. 2006 Practical endocrinology and diabetes in children, 2nd edn. Blackwell, Oxford

Puberty

Kalantaridou SN, Chrousos GP 2002 Clinical review 148: monogenic disorders of puberty. J Clin Endocrinol Metab 87: 2481–2494

Partsch CJ, Heger S, Sippell WG 2002 Management and outcome of central precocious puberty. Clin Endocrinol (Oxf) 56: 129–148

Disorders of sexual differentiation

Ahmed SF, Hughes IA 2002 The genetics of male undermasculinization. Clin Endocrinol (Oxf) 56: 1–18

Ahmed SF, Morrison S, Hughes IA 2004 Intersex and gender assignment: the third way? Arch Dis Child 89: 847–850

Hughes IA, Houk C, Ahmed SF et al. for the LWPES Consensus Group and ESPE Consensus Group 2006 Consensus statement on management of intersex disorders. Arch Dis Child 91: 554–563

Ogilvy-Stuart AL, Brain CE 2004 Early assessment of ambiguous genitalia. Arch Dis Child 89: 401–407

Transition of young people into adult services

Clayton PE, Cuneo RC, Juul A et al. for the European Society of Paediatric Endocrinology 2005 Consensus statement on the management of the GH-treated adolescent in the transition to adult care. Eur J Endocrinol 152: 165–170

Savage MO, Drake WM, Carroll PV et al. 2004 Transitional care of GH deficiency: when to stop GH therapy. Eur J Endocrinol 151(suppl 1): S61–S65

UK Department of Health 2006 National service framework for children, young people and maternity services. Transition: getting it right for young people. Improving the transition of young people with long-term conditions from children's to adult health services. UK Department of Health, London

SELF-ASSESSMENT

A 16-year-old male presents to the adult endocrine clinic. He is concerned that he is short and is embarrassed about changing in front of his peers. He is otherwise well. His mother experienced menarche at 16 years. Examination reveals that he is at pubic hair stage 1 and genital stage 1, with testicular volumes of 5 mL. His height is 153.1 cm. His LHRH test demonstrates basal and stimulated values of less than 0.1 and 3.6 U/L for FSH and 0.6 and 4.1 U/L for LH, respectively, and a basal testosterone level of 2.9 nmol/L.

Questions
1. What other information should be obtained?
2. What other investigations are needed?
3. What intervention is required?

Answers
1. See Boxes 2.3 and 2.11. Specific enquiry as to symptoms of chronic disease. The boy's height needs to be plotted on a growth chart and in the context of his parents' heights. There should be questioning as to whether there is a family history of delayed puberty, as is the case here.
2. In a well individual with a normal examination and a family history of delayed puberty, there is no need for any investigations at this stage. The clinical examination demonstrates that the patient is not prepubertal. Given the history and examination, the most likely diagnosis is CDGP. The LHRH test should not have been performed, and the result is compatible with his pubertal stage. Even though this test suggests hypogonadotrophic hypogonadism, the clinical examination suggests otherwise. The important point here is that the patient requires careful follow-up to ensure that he progresses through puberty and has not had a pubertal arrest. Accurate auxology will be required to evaluate his subsequent growth. If there is no pubertal progression, he should have the investigations detailed in Box 2.12 and the result of these should be checked prior to proceeding to an LHRH test.
3. The boy is significantly concerned about his appearance in terms of his height and stage of virilization. It should be explained that there is clinical evidence that he *has* entered puberty, albeit later than normal, and he would be expected to progress through puberty without any intervention. Also, his growth pattern is similar to his mother's. If he remains concerned, he should be offered testosterone injections (usually given as monthly 50-mg Sustanon injections for 4 months only). At follow-up visits, his auxology should be documented. In particular, a further increase in testicular volume would be expected, suggesting gonadotrophin release. If this does not occur, an alternative diagnosis should be considered and the patient should be discussed with a paediatric endocrinologist.

Disorders of the thyroid gland

3

L. D. K. E. Premawardhana and J. H. Lazarus

PHYSIOLOGY

The fetal thyroid gland begins developing during the fourth week of intrauterine life; this process involves cell differentiation and migration to its adult site, regulated by transcription factors PAX-8, FOXE-1 and NKX2.1. Follicles are identifiable by the 10th week, and hormone production commences around the 12th week. Therefore the developing fetus depends on maternal thyroid hormones during the crucial time of organogenesis before its own thyroid becomes fully functional. Thyroid follicles are lined by a single layer of cells surrounding colloid, which contains thyroglobulin, the template for thyroid hormone synthesis. The interfollicular spaces contain connective tissue, blood vessels and C cells that secrete calcitonin.

Hormone synthesis requires iodine that, after conversion to iodide, is concentrated in the thyroid (see Fig. 3.1). The sodium iodide symporter controls iodide uptake. Oxidized iodide then combines with thyroglobulin, stimulated by thyroid peroxidase to form monoiodotyrosine and diiodotyrosine. The coupling of two molecules of diiodotyrosine gives rise to thyroxine (T_4), and monoiodotyrosine with diiodotyrosine to triiodothyronine (T_3); these are then released to the circulation after proteolytic digestion of thyroglobulin. Thyroid-stimulating hormone (TSH) controls several steps in this process. T_4 and T_3 are conveyed to target tissues bound to transport proteins such as thyroxine-binding globulin (60–70%), transthyretin (15%), albumin (15–25%) and lipoproteins (very small amounts bound to high-density lipoprotein). Tissue accessibility is limited to the unbound fraction of thyroid hormone (free T_4 and free T_3).

The metabolic effects of thyroid hormones are mediated by free T_3 converted from T_4 by deiodinases (only 5–10% of circulating free T_3 is secreted by the thyroid). Free T_3 binds to nuclear hormone receptors (thyroid hormone receptor α_1 and thyroid hormone receptors β_1 and β_2), which act on response elements controlling gene expression. In addition to these genomic actions, thyroid hormones have also been reported to exert non-genomic effects, for example in the regulation of ion channels and mitochondrial function. Thyroid dysfunction may occur if any of the above mechanisms is defective (Table 3.1).

Figure 3.1
Iodine from food and iodinated compounds is trapped and transported through the thyrocyte into the follicular lumen. Oxidation and iodination of tyrosine residues of thyroglobulin occur in the colloid, giving rise to monoiodotyrosine and diiodotyrosine. Subsequent coupling of monoiodotyrosine and diiodotyrosine results in T_3 and T_4 formation, followed by proteolysis and release into the circulation. NIS – sodium iodide symporter; Tg – thyroglobulin; I – iodine; MIT – monoiodotyrosine; DIT – diiodotyrosine.

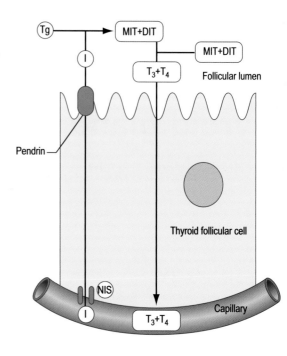

Table 3.1: Gene defects and thyroid dysfunction

Abnormality	Gene defect	Clinical features	Basis
Iodide transport	Sodium iodide symporter	Goitre, hypothyroidism	Reduced thyroid iodide levels
Iodide organification	Pendrin	Goitre, deafness	Reduced hormones
	Thyroglobulin, thyroid peroxidase	Goitre, hypothyroidism	
Deiodination of iodotyrosines	Deiodinase	Goitre, hypothyroidism	Reduced intrathyroidal iodine from monoiodotyrosine and diiodotyrosine
Hormone binding in serum	Thyroxine-binding globulin, transthyretin	Euthyroid	Reduced total thyroxine
	Albumin		Increased total thyroxine
Hormone action	Thyroid hormone β receptor	Variable clinical features	Resistance to thyroid hormone action
Hormone action and thyroid growth	TSH receptor:		
	• gain of function (germline)	Goitre, thyrotoxicosis	Constitutive activation of TSHR
	• gain of function (somatic)	Toxic adenoma	
	• loss of function	Hypothyroidism	TSH resistance

TSH, thyroid-stimulating hormone.

THYROID INVESTIGATIONS

Biochemical tests

Thyroid-stimulating hormone and free T_4 are common first-line tests in patients with suspected thyroid dysfunction.

Thyroid-stimulating hormone

Measurement of TSH (using a highly sensitive assay) is a good screening test in appropriate circumstances. It is very sensitive to free thyroid hormone activity and provides the earliest indication of thyroid dysfunction. However, measuring TSH alone would be inappropriate in:

- suspected pituitary–hypothalamic disease
- acute psychiatric disease or acutely ill in-patients (sick euthyroid or non-thyroidal illness syndrome; see later)
- the first trimester of pregnancy (low TSH caused by human chorionic gonadotrophin).

Free thyroxine and free triiodothyronine

Assays of free T_4 have replaced 'total' hormone activity. This removes the effects of factors such as the binding globulins. Assays of free T_3 in addition may be indicated in patients on liothyronine therapy or with amiodarone-induced thyrotoxicosis and when free T_4 is normal in suspected or treated thyrotoxicosis.

Thyroid autoantibodies

Antibodies to thyroglobulin, thyroid peroxidase and thyrotrophin receptors (both stimulating and blocking) are well characterized and clinically useful. Thyroid peroxidase antibodies have greater sensitivity than thyroglobulin antibodies and are used in preference to thyroglobulin antibodies in the diagnosis of autoimmune thyroid disease. Antibody assays (see Table 3.2) are now routinely available and will become less

Table 3.2: Indications for measuring thyroid autoantibodies

Thyroid antibody	Indication
Thyroid peroxidase antibody	Hashimoto's thyroiditis Postpartum thyroid disease Autoimmune polyglandular syndrome Pregnancy
Thyrotrophin receptor antibody	Graves' disease Neonatal hyperthyroidism Euthyroid ophthalmopathy

expensive in the future. About 10% of euthyroid female patients are thyroid peroxidase antibody or thyroglobulin antibody-positive.

Thyroid imaging

Chest x-ray

Views of the chest and neck may reveal retrosternal goitre and tracheal deviation and/or compression (see Figure 3.2).

Ultrasound

Ultrasound scans may be useful (although not routinely indicated) in:

- identifying and monitoring thyroid nodules
- guiding fine-needle aspiration cytology (FNAC)
- aspiration of cysts
- detecting autoimmune thyroid disease (e.g. the changes of hypoechogenicity of Hashimoto's disease and postpartum thyroiditis).

Colour flow Doppler sonography may be useful in amiodarone-induced thyrotoxicosis, although this is not widely used at present.

Radionuclide scans

Technetium and iodine scans are neither very sensitive nor specific. FNAC has superseded scanning in suspected thyroid tumours. The inability of malignant tissue to organify iodine results in the appearance of 'cold' nodules, and up to 20% of these may be

Figure 3.2
Chest x-ray showing retrosternal goitre.

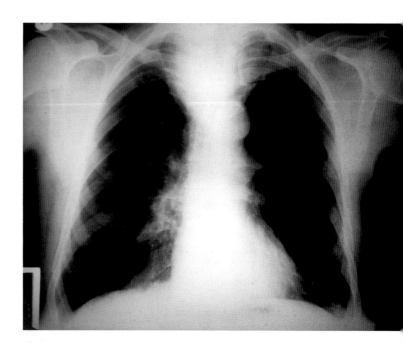

malignant. 'Warm' or 'hot' nodules signify only a less than 4% probability of malignancy. Radioactive iodine (RAI) uptake scans may be useful in:

- the differential diagnosis of thyrotoxicosis, uptake being low in destructive (e.g. subacute, postpartum, iodine and amiodarone-induced type 2 thyroiditis) and factitious thyrotoxicosis
- assessing dosimetry of ablative RAI
- assessing remnant thyroid activity after surgery for thyroid cancer
- diagnosing the cause of T_3 toxicosis (e.g. a toxic adenoma).

Computerized tomography and magnetic resonance imaging scans

Computerized tomography (CT) and magnetic resonance imaging (MRI) scans may be useful in assessing retrosternal goitres and tumours.

Fine-needle aspiration cytology of the thyroid gland

Fine-needle aspiration cytology, done under ultrasound guidance if required, is the method of choice in assessing thyroid nodules. It is safe (even in patients on aspirin or anticoagulants), easily performed and produces few complications. FNAC has reduced the need for surgery by almost 50% in the USA.

Fine-needle aspiration cytology is carried out using a 25-gauge needle attached to a plastic syringe (many operators use a syringe holder for ease of use). The patient is positioned supine with the neck extended (Fig. 3.3), and discouraged from talking or

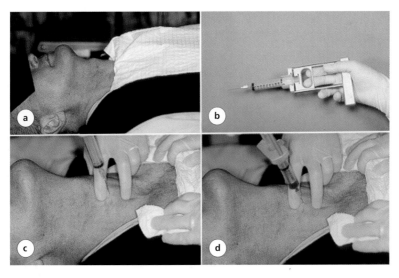

Figure 3.3
(a) Patient position for fine-needle aspiration cytology: supine, with the pillow under the patient's shoulder to allow hyperextension of the neck and maximal exposure. **(b)** Place the syringe in the syringe holder. **(c)** Standing on the side of the patient opposite that of the thyroid nodule, identify and stabilize the nodule with the 'non-aspirating' hand. **(d)** With a quick motion, pass the needle through the skin to enter the nodule. Immediate mild suction follows. As soon as aspirate appears, the suction is released and the needle withdrawn. (From Thyroid Disease Manager. Thyroid function tests. Online. Available: http://www.thyroidmanager.org/FunctionTests/fnabiopsy-frame.htm, courtesy of Leslie De Groot.)

swallowing during the procedure. After the nodule requiring aspiration is identified, the overlying skin is cleaned with alcohol. The needle is inserted into the nodule and suction applied and maintained while moving the needle back and forth within the nodule. When blood or fluid appears in the hub of the needle, suction is released and the needle should be withdrawn. A drop of the aspirated material should then be placed on a clean glass slide and, using a second glass slide, smears should be prepared and fixed in 95% alcohol in preparation for staining. Two to four such aspirations should be done for each nodule. Pressure is applied to the biopsy site after the procedure, and patients require observation for only a few minutes before discharge.

Indications for FNAC include:

- single nodule
- rapid enlargement or change in consistency of a nodule or nodules of a multinodular goitre
- localized thyroid abnormality in a Graves' or Hashimoto's goitre
- rapid growth of a diffuse goitre in middle-aged or elderly patients (to exclude lymphoma or anaplastic carcinoma).

The results of FNAC show:

- clearly benign cytology in about 70%
- clearly malignant cytology in 1–18%
- an inadequate sample in 5–10%
- indeterminate cytology in 15–20% (of which 10–30% are malignant at surgery).

Figure 3.4 shows an FNAC specimen from a patient with papillary carcinoma.

A higher yield of malignancy may be obtained in the future by using genetic markers of malignancy (e.g. B-RAF mutations) and other cellular markers (thyroid peroxidase or

Figure 3.4
Fine-needle aspiration cytology specimen from a patient with papillary carcinoma.

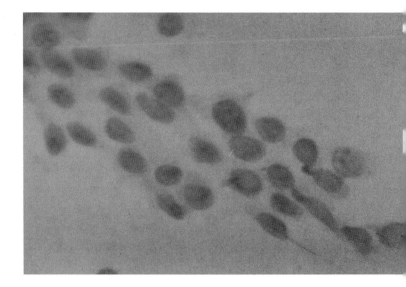

galectin-3). Those with malignant or indeterminate cytology should have surgery. The inability to distinguish between benign and malignant follicular lesions on cytology remains a problem.

THYROTOXICOSIS

An excess of thyroid hormones may be due to one of several mechanisms (Table 3.3). Graves' disease (70%), toxic multinodular goitre and toxic adenoma account for about 95% of cases.

Graves' disease

Graves' disease is the commonest form of thyrotoxicosis in iodine-sufficient areas. It affects relatively young women (average age 30–50 years) five to ten times more commonly than males, and they have a higher incidence of other autoimmune diseases (potentially shared genetic susceptibilities). It occurs due to the interaction of genetic predisposition and environmental factors. Familial aggregation (50%), concordance in twins (35–70% in monozygotic twins) and genetic polymorphisms in affected individuals suggest an important role for genetic factors. HLA D3 (in Caucasians) and cytotoxic T-lymphocyte antigen-4 polymorphisms contribute about 50% of the genetic susceptibility. Despite extensive candidate gene and genome-wide screens, no new susceptibility genes have emerged, although the thyroglobulin gene locus is promising.

Table 3.3: Causes of thyrotoxicosis

Diagnosis	Mechanism(s)
Graves' disease[a]	Thyroid-stimulating receptor antibody
Toxic multinodular goitre[a]	Excess iodine in previous multinodular goitre, ?thyroid-stimulating immunoglobulins
Toxic adenoma[a]	Activating TSH receptor mutations
Iodine-induced	Excessive iodine ingestion
Drug-induced	Amiodarone, lithium, radiocontrast media
Postpartum thyroiditis	Transient immune-mediated destruction
Subacute thyroiditis	Viral-induced destruction
Hyperemesis gravidarum	Human chorionic gonadotrophin-induced
Molar pregnancy	Human chorionic gonadotrophin-induced
Thyrotoxicosis factitia	Exogenous thyroid hormones
Pituitary resistance to thyroid hormone	Thyroid hormone β receptor mutation
Pituitary adenoma	Autonomous TSH secretion
Struma ovarii	Ectopic thyroid hormone production
Metastatic differentiated thyroid cancer	Ectopic thyroid hormone production
Hereditary hyperthyroidism (autosomal dominant)	Constitutive TSH receptor activation
Silent thyroiditis	Lymphocytic infiltration

TSH, thyroid-stimulating hormone.
[a]The three most common causes of thyrotoxicosis.

Several environmental factors precipitating Graves' disease have also been identified.

- Excess iodine: the Jod–Basedow effect, altered immunogenicity or release of antigens. (The replenishing of iodine stores in individuals who are predisposed to autoimmune thyroid disease but were previously lacking iodine may induce thyrotoxicosis – this is the Jod–Basedow effect.)
- Interferon-α: effects on immunoregulatory mechanisms.
- Smoking: major risk factor for ophthalmopathy (hypoxia increases synthesis of orbital glycosaminoglycans).
- Anti-CD52 antibody: conversion of a Th1 (interferon-γ-dominated) to a proinflammatory Th2 (interleukin-4-dominated) phenotype. Anti-CD52 is a Th2 inducer favouring antibody-mediated immunity.

The mediators of Graves' disease are stimulatory thyrotrophin receptor antibodies, which are found in over 90% of patients with Graves' disease. Thyroid peroxidase antibodies (75–80%) and thyroglobulin antibodies (25–55%, usually in low titre) may also be found.

The clinical features of Graves' hyperthyroidism are common to other forms of thyrotoxicosis. Graves' orbitopathy (30–50%), pretibial myxoedema (5%) and thyroid acropachy (<1%) occur in a minority.

Diagnosis of Graves' disease

On confirmation of biochemical thyrotoxicosis, thyrotrophin receptor antibodies, thyroid peroxidase antibodies and – if indicated (e.g. to differentiate from destructive thyroiditis) – RAI uptake scanning (diffuse increase in uptake) may be used to confirm Graves' disease and to exclude other causes (Fig. 3.5).

Figure 3.5
Biochemical diagnosis of thyrotoxicosis. FT$_3$, free triiodothyronine; FT$_4$, free thyroxine; T$_3$, triiodothyronine; TSH, thyroid-stimulating hormone.

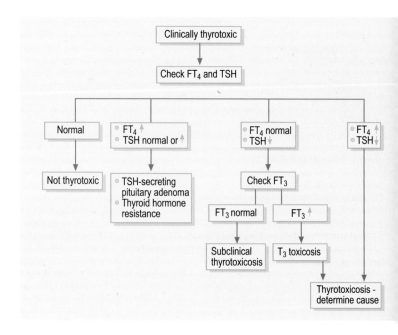

Management of Graves' disease

Antithyroid drugs (carbimazole and propylthiouracil), RAI and surgery may be used alone or in combination. Antithyroid drugs are first-line therapy in the majority of patients during a first episode of Graves' disease (see Table 3.4).

The choice of regimen (block and replacement versus titration) and duration of therapy are still matters for debate. A recent systematic review of 23 randomized controlled trials concluded that there was no difference in relapse rates at 2–5 years when the two regimens were compared, but minor and major side-effects and withdrawals from treatment were marginally more common in the block and replacement regimen. None of the trials examined the issue of transient hypothyroidism on quality of life and progression of ophthalmopathy (very often arguments advanced in favour of the block and replacement regimen). When different titration regimens were compared, there was no difference in relapse rates between the 12- versus 24- and 24- versus 42-month regimens, respectively. There was also no benefit from the addition of T_4 after a course of antithyroid drugs. Caution needs to be exercised when interpreting these data, as there was a very high dropout rate from all the studies considered in this review. However, of those medically treated only about 40–50% are in remission at 10 years.

Antithyroid drugs may produce minor side-effects, which include skin reactions, arthralgia and transient migratory polyarthritis. Gastrointestinal upsets occur in a minority. Antihistamines may be required for skin eruptions while the antithyroid drug is continued or changed to a different group (although cross-reactivity occurs in about 50%). Antithyroid drugs may need to be stopped if severe reactions occur, and early RAI therapy should be considered in these patients.

Table 3.4: Medical treatment of Graves' disease

Drug(s)	Regimen[a]
Carbimazole, methimazole, propylthiouracil[b]	**Titration regimen:** • start carbimazole 40 mg/day (or equivalent doses of methimazole) or propylthiouracil, 400–450 mg/day • reduce gradually to maintain euthyroidism (carbimazole 5–10 mg/day) • continue for 12–18 months **Block and replacement regimen:** • carbimazole 40 mg/day or propylthiouracil 150 mg t.d.s. • add thyroxine 100–150 µg/day when euthyroid (3–6 weeks) • continue for 6–9 months
Propranolol	20–80 mg t.d.s. to block sympathetic features in the initial few weeks

[a]Carbimazole appears to have a slightly better side-effect profile. With the titration regimen, a 12- to 18-month course of therapy appears better (fewer relapses) than shorter or longer courses. A 6-month block and replacement regimen appears to be no less effective than a 12-month course. Recurrences are commonest in the first year after stopping treatment. The block and replacement regimen using high doses of carbimazole/methimazole is not recommended in pregnancy, because of the risk of inducing fetal hypothyroidism and goitre. Propylthiouracil is preferred in pregnancy, because there is no reported risk of aplasia cutis and embryopathy (which rarely occur with carbimazole/methimazole).
[b]Written warning or documented verbal instructions of serious side-effects should be issued to all patients.

Agranulocytosis (a granulocyte count of $<0.5 \times 10^9$/L), which is probably immune-mediated, is fortunately rare (0.37% for propylthiouracil and 0.35% for carbimazole). It usually occurs in the first 3 months but may occur late and during a second course of antithyroid drugs. A white cell count is often measured before treatment is commenced, but there is no consensus about the utility of periodic neutrophil counts to predict agranulocytosis. Patients should be warned to seek urgent medical attention if fever and sore throat occur. Antithyroid drugs should be stopped and appropriate in-hospital intravenous antibiotic therapy (to include cover for *Pseudomonas*) should be commenced immediately. Haematologists should be involved early in management to advise about granulocyte colony-stimulating factor therapy and bone marrow aspiration. The management of thyrotoxicosis in these patients may require unconventional modes of therapy (e.g. lithium), as there is some cross-sensitivity between carbimazole and propylthiouracil.

Propylthiouracil rarely causes an allergic hepatitis associated with a poor prognosis. In this instance, propylthiouracil should be withdrawn and liver failure managed in a specialized unit. This type of liver dysfunction should be differentiated from the more common, benign and transient liver enzyme increase (up to six times normal), which is self-limiting despite continued therapy. Cholestatic liver dysfunction may occur with carbimazole and methimazole but recovers on drug withdrawal. In the above situations, the careful introduction of the alternative class of antithyroid or other drugs may have to be considered.

Antithyroid drugs, particularly propylthiouracil, may also cause a vasculitis (some antineutrophil cytoplasmic antibody-positive) with multisystem involvement. Immediate drug withdrawal (with remission in most), high-dose glucocorticoids, cyclophosphamide and haemodialysis may be required.

The use of lithium and perchlorate to reduce hormone secretion is limited by side-effects. Iodine and amiodarone are only rarely used, and cholestyramine may be combined with carbimazole or propylthiouracil occasionally to reduce hormone levels quicker. Half of all patients with thyrotoxicosis-induced atrial fibrillation revert to sinus rhythm when euthyroid, and the rest should be cardioverted. Warfarin (or aspirin if warfarin is contraindicated) should be considered in all of them, as the risk of thromboembolism is increased in these patients.

Radioiodine therapy is used in patients with recurrent disease and in the elderly (increasingly as first-line therapy), and 5–20% may require a second dose. About 10–20% of RAI-treated patients become hypothyroid in the first year and 5–10% per year thereafter, although this is dependent on the dose of RAI given, and higher rates may be encountered if the policy within a unit is to ablate the thyroid. Antithyroid drugs may be needed in severe thyrotoxicosis (particularly in the elderly) to achieve clinical and biochemical euthyroidism before RAI and for 3–4 weeks thereafter (antithyroid drugs need to be stopped for 3–4 days before and 2–3 days after RAI). RAI is definitely contraindicated during pregnancy and breast feeding. Thyroid-associated ophthalmopathy is a relative contraindication. However, in non-sight-threatening disease, prednisolone 30–40 mg/day given for 1 month after RAI and gradually reduced thereafter prevents deterioration of ophthalmopathy. Patients should be warned to avoid conception for 6–12 months. Men may have a reduced sperm count for up to 2 years after treatment. Close contact with young children (within less than 1 m according to current advice) should be avoided for several weeks, depending on the dose of RAI given. Patients should avoid travel by public transport (to protect others from irradiation) and warned to carry their radiation certificate if travelling by air (as there is a risk of setting off sensitive airport security alarms). Long-term hypothyroidism is possible, and patients should be warned of the need for T_4 treatment if this occurs. There is no long-term risk of cancer.

Surgery is reserved for patients with suspicious lesions, for those unwilling or unable to have RAI or for those with a personal cosmetic preference. Patients should be rendered clinically and biochemically euthyroid prior to surgery.

Toxic multinodular goitre

Multiple autonomous nodules produce excess thyroid hormones in toxic multinodular goitre, a condition that is more common in elderly women and in iodine-deficient areas. Symptoms are similar to those of other forms of thyrotoxicosis, but cardiac symptoms often predominate because of the age of affected patients. Graves' orbitopathy, pretibial myxoedema and acropachy do not occur. Large retrosternal goitres may occasionally cause pressure symptoms. Free T_4, TSH and RAI uptake scans, if necessary (multiple hot and cold areas), help establish the diagnosis. The majority of these patients are thyroid peroxidase antibody-negative. RAI is the preferred therapy, preceded by antithyroid drugs. Goitres producing pressure symptoms and suspicious nodules may require surgery.

Toxic adenoma

A single hyperfunctioning nodule occurs in 5% of thyrotoxic patients. In some, TSH receptor and Gs alpha gene mutations stimulate growth and function, leading to clonal expansion and nodule formation. Clinical and biochemical features are similar to those of toxic multinodular goitre, although isolated T_3 thyrotoxicosis is particularly common in toxic adenomas. RAI uptake scans reveal a hot nodule (with suppression elsewhere). RAI is the treatment of choice, and surgery is reserved for large or suspicious nodules, particularly in young patients.

Subclinical hyperthyroidism

Subclinical hyperthyroidism is characterized by low or undetectable TSH and normal free T_3 and free T_4. The causes of subclinical hyperthyroidism are similar to those of overt hyperthyroidism. In addition, about 20% of hypothyroid patients on T_4 treatment are also affected. It is important to recognize that low or undetectable TSH may be a feature of pituitary–hypothalamic disease, non-thyroidal illness syndrome or drug therapy (e.g. glucocorticoids) and should be investigated appropriately. The incidence of subclinical hyperthyroidism is unknown, but prevalence rates of up to 16% have been quoted.

It should be noted that TSH normalizes without intervention in nearly 50% with endogenous disease (Graves' disease, toxic multinodular goitre or toxic adenoma). Overt hyperthyroidism develops more commonly in patients with undetectable TSH.

Several cardiovascular (tachycardia, atrial fibrillation, systolic and diastolic dysfunction), bone (conflicting evidence about reduced mineral density and fracture) and quality of life issues have been linked to subclinical hyperthyroidism.

Regular monitoring and dose adjustment in patients on T_4 replacement or suppressive T_4 therapy, combined if necessary with beta blockade and bisphosphonates, may prevent the effects of exogenous subclinical hyperthyroidism. Patients with endogenous disease (especially those who are elderly and at risk of osteoporosis and cardiac disease) whose TSH levels are completely suppressed may require specific antithyroid therapy. However, there are no firm guidelines.

THYROIDITIS

This group of inflammatory disorders is characterized by lymphocytic cell infiltration and fibrosis. Several distinct clinical conditions occur.

Acute thyroiditis

Bacterial, fungal and rarely parasitic infection causes neck pain, tenderness, skin redness and swelling. Patients complain of dysphagia, and there may be symptoms of pharyngitis and fever. Thyroid hormones and RAI uptake are usually normal, but FNAC provides microbiological proof and guidance to therapy.

Subacute (de Quervain's) thyroiditis

Probably of viral origin, this condition is more common in females. It is often preceded by a viral or respiratory prodrome, and systemic symptoms are common. Abrupt onset of neck pain, high erythrocyte sedimentation rate and low RAI uptake (destructive thyroiditis) aid diagnosis. An initial thyrotoxic phase due to release of preformed hormone, requiring beta blocker therapy occasionally, is usually followed by a transient hypothyroid phase sometimes requiring T_4 therapy. Eventual recovery occurs in most between 6 and 12 months. Aspirin and non-steroidal anti-inflammatory drugs relieve the pain and malaise, but glucocorticoids may occasionally be needed and produce both rapid and dramatic improvement in symptoms.

Subacute lymphocytic thyroiditis

Clinically similar to de Quervain's thyroiditis (although painless), this self-limiting condition occurs spontaneously or postpartum and is similarly managed (see later).

Riedel's thyroiditis

This rare, fibrotic disorder involves the thyroid and surrounding structures and may produce tracheal and oesophageal obstruction. A hard goitre is found in middle-aged or elderly women who are euthyroid or rarely hypothyroid. Fibrosis may occur elsewhere, producing mediastinitis, retroperitoneal and retro-orbital fibrosis and sclerosing cholangitis. About half of these patients are thyroid antibody-positive. Surgical biopsy is needed for diagnosis. Wedge resection of the isthmus, steroids and tamoxifen may be tried.

GRAVES' ORBITOPATHY

Graves' orbitopathy develops in 25–50% of patients with Graves' disease, and 3–5% of these may suffer severe and sight-threatening disease.

Risk factors

Graves' orbitopathy is more likely in current or former smokers than in those who have never smoked, and stopping smoking reduces the risk. Women have a higher risk of Graves' orbitopathy because of their higher incidence of Graves' disease. RAI therapy may cause transient worsening of existing Graves' orbitopathy, and steroids are used in its prevention (see previous sections).

Pathogenesis

The pathogenesis of Graves' orbitopathy remains unclear, but a link with thyrotrophin receptor antibodies is now emerging. The TSH receptor is a shared antigen between the thyroid gland, orbital tissue and skin (in patients with pretibial myxoedema). Although thyrotrophin receptor antibody activity correlates with Graves' orbitopathy severity, its specific role in Graves' orbitopathy remains unproven. There is emerging evidence to suggest a role also for activated T lymphocytes, which are found in abundance in the orbits of affected patients. Inflammatory cytokines derived from these cause preadipocyte differentiation, fibroblast proliferation and glycosaminoglycan production, all of which are features of Graves' orbitopathy.

Clinical features

The clinical features and severity of Graves' orbitopathy may be classified using clinical signs only (NO SPECS classification) or symptoms and signs of disease activity (pain, redness, swelling and impaired function). These help in monitoring and planning intervention.

The clinical features of Graves' orbitopathy may include:

- lid lag and retraction (50%)
- periorbital oedema, tearing and grittiness (40%) (Fig. 3.6)

Figure 3.6
Periorbital oedema, chemosis and limitation of upwards gaze in a patient with Graves' orbitopathy.

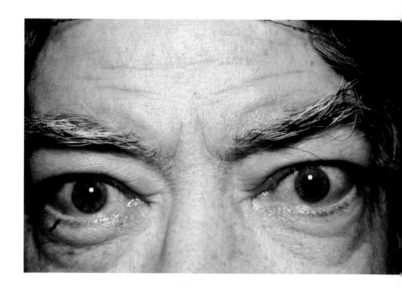

- proptosis (30%)
- muscle dysfunction – diplopia looking upwards and outwards (10%)
- exposure keratitis (<5%)
- optic nerve compression and blindness (<1%).

Urgent ophthalmic referral is indicated if optic nerve involvement is suspected: blurred vision, impaired colour perception, reduced visual acuity, afferent papillary defects or visual field loss.

Diagnostic pitfalls

Diagnostic pitfalls are as follows.

- The absence of features of thyrotoxicosis. About 10% of patients with Graves' orbitopathy are euthyroid and 10% hypothyroid at presentation. Investigations should include CT/MRI of the orbits (to demonstrate extraocular muscle swelling with tendon sparing), thyrotrophin receptor antibody and thyroid peroxidase antibody activity, and tests of thyroid function.
- Unilateral signs. About 10% have unilateral signs. CT/MRI scans of the orbit show contralateral eye muscle involvement in 50–90% of them. The differential diagnosis includes orbital tumours (lymphoma, glioma, meningioma, rhabdomyosarcoma, haemangioma and metastases), orbital myositis and cellulitis, granulomatous disease (sarcoidosis and Wegener granulomatosis) and cavernous sinus thrombosis. Relevant investigations should be done if there is a clinical suspicion. Rarely, orbital biopsy may be indicated.

Management of Graves' orbitopathy

The management of Graves' orbitopathy is ideally done in a combined thyroid and ophthalmology clinic. The majority of patients require only symptom relief with artificial tears, eye protection and advice about sleeping propped up. In the minority requiring intervention, early treatment (while ophthalmopathy is active) produces the best results. Smoking should be actively discouraged, as it delays and diminishes the effects of medical treatment. High-dose steroids (oral prednisolone 60–120 mg/day with or without steroid-sparing agents, or an infusion of high-dose steroids for 3 days) and/or orbital radiotherapy may be required in 10–35% of patients with sight-threatening disease, anterior congestive changes, worsening diplopia and optic nerve compression. Steroids may benefit 33–66% of these patients. Orbital radiotherapy may be considered in those without diabetic or hypertensive retinopathy, although this remains controversial. In those who have active disease and who respond poorly to medical therapy, surgical orbital decompression may be required. Surgery may also be indicated for cosmetic reasons and functional improvement in burnt-out disease. Cytokine antagonists, octreotide, colchicine and cyclosporin are agents currently being assessed.

PRIMARY HYPOTHYROIDISM

Hypothyroidism (see Box 3.1) affects 1.5–2% women and <1% men in the UK and USA. Clinical features are non-specific and too insensitive to be used alone in diagnosis. Cold intolerance, weight gain, dry skin, constipation, bradycardia and myotonic ankle jerks are common features, while galactorrhoea, menorrhagia and joint and pleuropericardial effusions are present only in a minority. TSH is a sensitive diagnostic test in primary hypothyroidism, but it is inappropriate in pituitary–hypothalamic hypothyroidism and in the thyroid hormone resistance syndromes.

Hashimoto's thyroiditis

The commonest form of hypothyroidism in Caucasians is Hashimoto's thyroiditis (iodine deficiency is a more common cause worldwide) due to autoimmune destruction and

---

Box 3.1: Causes of hypothyroidism

- Hashimoto's disease
- Radioiodine therapy
- Previous thyroidectomy
- Antithyroid drug therapy
- Postpartum thyroid disease (usually transient)
- Drugs
    Lithium
    Amiodarone
    Iodide
    Interferon-α
- Pituitary disease
- Hypothalamic disease
- Subacute or silent thyroiditis
- Iodine deficiency
- Generalized resistance to thyroid hormone

Table 3.5: Reversible causes of hypothyroidism

Diagnosis	Reversibility
Hashimoto's disease	About 5% recover due to decreasing thyroid-stimulating hormone receptor-blocking antibodies
Postpartum thyroiditis	Up to 70% recover in the first year
Subacute thyroiditis	Nearly 100% recover
Iodine-induced	The majority become normal when iodine excess is reduced
Drug-induced	The majority become normal when drugs are withdrawn
Post-ablative (surgery and radioactive iodine therapy)	Hypothyroidism may be temporary

lymphocytic infiltration of the thyroid. Extensive fibrosis prevents goitre formation in some patients (spontaneous atrophic thyroiditis). Thyroid peroxidase antibodies (>90%), thyroglobulin antibodies (5–25%) and TSH-blocking antibodies are found more commonly in female patients with this condition. Most symptoms are non-specific, as indicated above. Hashimoto's thyroiditis may occur in patients with Addison's disease (30%), type 1 diabetes mellitus (5–10%) and coeliac disease (5%). The presence of goitre, low free T_4 and high TSH, and thyroid antibodies establishes the diagnosis of Hashimoto's thyroiditis. Separate investigations may be needed to diagnose associated disorders. Although permanent hypothyroidism requires lifelong treatment, reversible causes for hypothyroidism (Table 3.5) need to be identified.

Occasionally, primary hypothyroidism is due to blocking thyrotrophin receptor antibodies; this may be reversible if antibody levels fall and there is sufficient capacity in the remaining gland for adequate thyroid hormone synthesis. Furthermore, a change in the nature of thyrotrophin receptor antibodies from blocking to stimulatory may induce Graves' thyrotoxicosis.

Management

Levothyroxine (LT_4), liothyronine and combinations of the two are available for replacement therapy, although it should be emphasized that combination therapy has not been shown to be superior to LT_4 alone. A recent meta-analysis failed to show a benefit for combination therapy over LT_4 monotherapy in terms of symptoms, quality of life, cognition, lipid profiles and weight in patients who had LT_4 monotherapy only and in patients who were given a combination because of dissatisfaction with monotherapy. The authors concluded that LT_4 should remain the standard treatment for hypothyroidism. The goals of replacement are normalization of TSH and symptom control. Starting doses of LT_4 should be small in patients with cardiac disease (e.g. 25–50 μg/day), with dose increases every 4–6 weeks. However, in young and otherwise healthy older patients LT_4 may be started at higher dosage (100 and 50 μg/day, respectively). Doses should be increased every 4–6 weeks if necessary. In patients suspected of having hypoadrenalism, glucocorticoid replacement should be started before LT_4 to prevent an acute hypoadrenal crisis. Persistently raised TSH levels may occur in patients on standard doses of LT_4.

> **Box 3.2: Causes of raised thyroid-stimulating hormone levels in hypothyroid patients on replacement levothyroxine**
>
> - Non-compliance with medication: supervised administration of standard dose or single weekly doses of 1000 μg may be tried
> - Inadequate dose: dispensing error, change in levothyroxine (LT$_4$) formulation
> - Interaction with other drugs
> - Reduced absorption: iron tablets, cholestyramine, calcium carbonate, soya
> - Rapid clearance of LT$_4$: phenytoin, carbamazepine, rifampin, valproate
> - Decreased function of residual gland tissue
> - Autoimmune thyroid disease, post irradiation
> - Pregnancy
> - Postmenopausal oestrogen treatment (increase in thyroxine-binding globulin levels)
> - Systemic illness
> - Development of malabsorption (e.g. coeliac disease)
> - Massive proteinuria in the nephrotic syndrome

Although this is most commonly due to poor compliance, other causes should be sought when compliance is assured, and LT$_4$ doses may need to be increased (Box 3.2).

Twenty per cent of patients on LT$_4$ therapy have suppressed TSH levels, a risk for osteoporosis (particularly in postmenopausal women). Close monitoring of thyroid function, with dose reduction of LT$_4$ if appropriate, is therefore recommended. T$_4$ dose increases should be anticipated in gluten sensitivity, pregnancy and drug therapy (Box 3.2). Altered bioavailability is reported when there is a change of T$_4$ formulation.

Subclinical hypothyroidism

The combination of elevated TSH with normal free T$_4$ and free T$_3$ is seen commonly. Subclinical hypothyroidism is more prevalent in the elderly and in women (17% in women and 7% in men over 65 years; 4–10% in the general population). TSH returns to normal in about 5% of these in 1 year. Progression to overt hypothyroidism depends on initial TSH and the presence of thyroid peroxidase antibodies and is estimated to occur at a rate of 5–5.5% per year.

Subclinical hypothyroidism may be caused by chronic autoimmune thyroid disease, surgery, RAI, antithyroid drugs, inadequate T$_4$ replacement, and subacute and postpartum thyroiditis. Clinical manifestations are minor and non-specific and associated with higher TSH levels. Somatic, neurocognitive and metabolic abnormalities are said to occur more commonly in subclinical hypothyroidism, but the evidence is currently inconclusive. A recent study showed aortic atherosclerosis and myocardial infarction occurring more commonly in elderly women with subclinical hypothyroidism, with a population attributable risk for myocardial infarction similar to other major risk factors.

Management

Transient hypothyroidism should be excluded by repeating the TSH in 4–12 weeks. LT$_4$ treatment should be given to patients with a TSH greater than 10 mU/L, as the evidence for improved outcomes (symptoms, depression, metabolic and cardiac) is more compelling in this group. Uncertainty remains about the treatment of patients with raised TSH levels below 10 mU/L; current recommendations are to monitor annually patients with TSH between 4.5 and 10 mU/L. A trial of T_4 therapy for 3–6 months may be undertaken in patients with significant symptoms, although only 25–30% show improvement. Current guidelines indicate that the presence of thyroid peroxidase antibodies should not influence intervention at any level of TSH (although progression to overt hypothyroidism is greater in thyroid peroxidase antibody-positive versus thyroid peroxidase antibody-negative patients: 4.3% versus 2.6% per year, respectively). However, pregnancy and/or its anticipation are indications for LT_4 therapy at all levels of raised TSH to prevent potential neurocognitive deficits in the offspring. It should be remembered that treatment does not alter the natural history of subclinical hypothyroidism.

SCREENING FOR THYROID DISEASE

Clinical features alone lack sensitivity and specificity in diagnosing thyroid dysfunction. Most authorities advocate a targeted aggressive case-finding strategy (using TSH), but universal screening, particularly of older subjects, is recommended by some. Screening may be beneficial in the following groups with a possible increased risk of thyroid dysfunction:

- previous thyroid disease/surgery or postpartum thyroid dysfunction
- goitre
- type 1 diabetes mellitus
- other autoimmune endocrine disease
- drug therapy (amiodarone, lithium, interferon-α, etc.)
- pituitary–hypothalamic disease
- polycystic ovary syndrome
- Down's syndrome
- Turner's syndrome
- head and neck irradiation
- primary pulmonary hypertension
- type 2 diabetes mellitus

(A definite link with increased risk is not proven in some of the above.) Thyroid testing may become standard practice in women planning pregnancy, but neonatal screening for congenital hypothyroidism is currently routine in many countries.

SICK EUTHYROID SYNDROME (NON-THYROIDAL ILLNESS SYNDROME)

Non-thyroidal illness (in the absence of primary thyroid or pituitary–hypothalamic disease; see Box 3.3) produces several effects on thyroid hormone activity. These effects

Box 3.3: Causes of non-thyroidal illness syndrome

- Myocardial infarction
- Pneumonia
- Sepsis, HIV, tuberculosis, malaria
- Chronic renal failure, nephritic syndrome
- Coronary artery bypass graft, transplant surgery, caesarean section
- Cirrhosis, hepatitis
- Diabetic ketoacidosis, starvation, malnutrition
- Depression
- Burns
- Malignancy

depend on the severity and duration of the illness rather than the specific illness, and the magnitude of change relates to its severity. Non-thyroidal illness syndrome is confirmed by a return to normal of these changes at recovery. The mechanisms causing non-thyroidal illness syndrome relate to altered hormone production, transport, distribution and metabolism and to pituitary TSH production. The acute changes are probably cytokine-mediated and mainly peripheral, but the changes of prolonged critical illness are mainly neuroendocrine. These effects are compounded by concomitant drug therapy.

The hormonal abnormalities are assay-dependent, but several patterns have been identified. Low total T_3 (40% of normal) and free T_3 (60% of normal) with normal free T_4 is the commonest and is seen in about 70% of acutely ill hospitalized patients. Low total T_4 levels are also often present in severely ill (and often moribund) patients in intensive care, indicating a poor prognosis. Some patients on dopamine and corticosteroids also have low free T_4 from TSH suppression. Patients with chronic liver disease and porphyria have a high total T_4 but normal free T_4 (probably due to raised thyroxine-binding globulin levels). Isolated TSH abnormalities (low and marginally elevated levels) are less common. Undetectable TSH levels in third-generation assays are due to intrinsic disease in over 70% of patients.

Thyroxine replacement does not improve outcome in critically ill patients, and high doses may be harmful (treatment in premature infants is still under review). However, replacement should continue in patients with known thyroid disease. If urgent treatment (suspected thyrotoxic crisis or myxoedema coma) is not indicated, it is safe to repeat thyroid tests after recovery before deciding on long-term treatment. Clinical evidence (goitre, ophthalmopathy, skin and nail changes), thyroid peroxidase antibody and RAI uptake scans may help in some patients. Suspicion of hypothalamic–pituitary disease indicates the need for appropriate investigations.

NODULAR THYROID DISEASE

Excessive growth of one or more areas of the thyroid produces a nodular goitre (Fig. 3.7). Hyperfunction of these nodules will in turn produce a toxic multinodular goitre or toxic adenoma (see above). In the absence of autoimmune thyroid disease,

Figure 3.7
Retrosternal goitre and subclavian venogram (with subtraction) showing its extent.

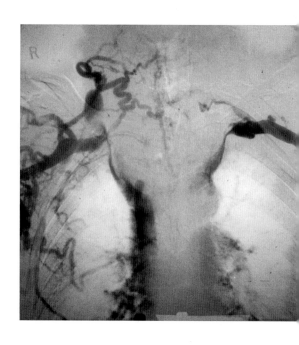

malignancy, thyroid dysfunction and thyroiditis, these goitres are called simple nodular goitres and may be endemic in iodine-deficient areas, or sporadic. Female gender, smoking, goitrogens (e.g. flavonoids and thiocyanates) and possibly stress and infection increase the risk of sporadic simple nodular goitres. Symptoms are related to neck swelling, thyrotoxicosis and tracheal (breathlessness, stridor) or oesophageal compression. Neck vein distension made worse by extending the arms above the head (Pemberton's sign), facial plethora and vocal cord paralysis may occur. At examination, risk factors for malignancy should be assessed (Table 3.6). Investigations including thyroid peroxidase antibodies, TSH, RAI uptake scans, FNAC and calcitonin assays (family history of thyroid cancer) may be needed. A flow volume loop and tracheal MRI may help in assessing the effects of compression.

The natural history of simple nodular goitres is variable and difficult to predict. Rates of growth between 4.5 and 20% have been estimated. Those that become toxic do so insidiously, and a long subclinical phase very often intervenes.

No uniform guidelines exist for the management of simple nodular goitres. T_4 therapy, if tried, needs to be lifelong, has a variable efficacy and is contraindicated when TSH is suppressed. At recommended TSH-suppressive doses, it may cause atrial fibrillation and bone effects in the predisposed. Surgery may be considered for symptom relief, for tracheal decompression, for goitre size reduction and for providing a histological diagnosis. However, there is a risk of recurrence (15–40%) and complications. RAI therapy may reduce goitre size by 50% at 1 year and may be repeated if necessary. Isolation may be needed after the higher doses required for large goitres (recombinant human TSH may reduce this), and long-term morbidity may occur in these patients. Solitary nodules may also be managed as above. Percutaneous ethanol injection and laser photocoagulation are currently experimental.

Thyroid incidentaloma

Impalpable thyroid nodules (<10 mm in diameter) are diagnosed more frequently at thyroid scanning and at surgery for unrelated reasons. FNAC should be undertaken in nodules more than 10 mm in diameter in view of a small but definite risk of malignancy (higher for solid, hypoechogenic nodules with irregular margins and microcalcification). Guidelines indicate that smaller nodules may safely be observed.

THYROID CANCER

Thyroid cancers are the commonest endocrine malignancy, with an incidence of 2.3 and 0.9 per 100000 in women and men, respectively. There are about 900 new cases and 220 deaths per year in England and Wales. A dramatic increase in aggressive cancers occurred in children exposed to radiation following the Chernobyl accident. The 10-year survival rates for papillary and follicular cancers were 93–94% and 84–85%, respectively, in large American studies. Recurrences, both local or regional (30%) and distant (20%), occur and increase with time. Increasing age and widespread metastases are associated with a poor prognosis (Box 3.4).

There are well-recognized but rare syndromes of familial thyroid cancers associated with tumours in other organs:

- Cowden syndrome (hamartomas; breast, colon and lung tumours)
- Gardner syndrome (intestinal polyps, osteomas, fibromas and lipomas)
- Carney complex (pigmented adrenal nodules, pituitary tumours, skin pigmentation and myxomas)
- Turcot syndrome (large intestinal polyps and brain tumours).

Histological types

Papillary thyroid carcinoma (PTC) accounts for about 80–85% of cancers in iodine-sufficient areas. RET/PTC mutations (leading to unregulated tyrosine kinase activation),

---

Box 3.4: Indicators of poor prognosis in thyroid cancer

- Extremes of age
- Male gender
- Poorly differentiated histology
- Advanced tumours
- Large tumours
- Extension beyond thyroid capsule
- Distant metastases (lymph node, haematogenous)
- Multifocality
- Inadequate surgical treatment and follow-up
- Incomplete resection
- Ablative radioiodine therapy not given
- Elevated serum thyroglobulin more than 3 months after surgery

B-RAF and RAS gene mutations are found in about 70% of these patients. Follicular carcinomas accounting for about 5–10% of cancers are commoner in iodine-deficient areas. Translocations of the DNA-binding domain of PAX-8 to the PPAR-γ1 gene have been identified in these tumours recently. Medullary thyroid carcinomas arising from C cells account for about 3–5%. Hurthle cell neoplasms, poorly differentiated cancers and undifferentiated (anaplastic) cancers are very uncommon. Primary lymphomas (usually occurring in patients with pre-existing Hashimoto's disease) and sarcomas are also very rare. Metastases to the thyroid may occur from the breast, colon, kidneys and melanomas but are extremely rare.

Clinical features and diagnosis

The clinical features suggesting an increased likelihood of malignancy in a single nodule are shown in Table 3.6.

Papillary carcinomas occur more commonly in females and in the 20- to 30-year age group. They may be multicentric and spread locally to involve cervical and mediastinal lymph nodes. Occasionally, spread may occur to the lungs. Long-term survival is excellent but may be adversely affected by age (over 45 years), extrathyroidal spread and tumour size (over 3 cm).

Follicular carcinomas occur in older individuals (the fifth decade) and are more common in women. Distant metastases (to lung and bone) are more common than local lymphatic spread and may be in 50% at diagnosis. Long-term survival is worse than in papillary tumours.

Undifferentiated carcinomas usually occur in individuals over the age of 50 years and may sometimes arise in previously benign lesions or in known differentiated cancers. Aggressive local (trachea or oesophagus), regional and distal lymphatic and haematogenous spread (to the lungs) is common. Survival beyond 6 months to 1 year is rare.

Table 3.6: Clinical features and likelihood of malignancy in a single nodule

Clinical feature	Likelihood of malignancy
Rapid growth	High
Firm or hard consistency	High
Attachment to surrounding structures	High
Lymph node involvement	High
Metastases	High
Vocal cord involvement	High
Family history of multiple endocrine neoplasia or medullary thyroid carcinoma	High
Extremes of age (<20 or >70 years)	Moderate
Male	Moderate
Large nodule (>4 cm)	Moderate
History of head/neck irradiation	Moderate
Symptoms of compression	Moderate

Diagnosis is established in most instances by FNAC (sensitivity >90%). RAI uptake scans are not routinely indicated (but if done may identify 'cold nodules', 20% of which may be malignant). There are several staging systems in use, such as:

- the tumour, node, metastasis (TNM) system (incorporating the American Joint Committee on Cancer, AJCC, staging scheme)
- the European Organization for Research and Treatment of Cancer system
- the DAMES system
- the distant metastasis, patient age, completeness of resection, local invasion and tumour size (MACIS) system.

These systems broadly separate low- and high-risk groups.

Management

Total or near-total thyroidectomy (all visible thyroid tissue is removed except for a small amount near the insertion of the recurrent laryngeal nerve) is recommended for differentiated cancers. Subtotal and hemithyroidectomy are out of favour, because a significant number of thyroid tumours are multicentric and bilateral. Completion thyroidectomy may be needed in patients who have had incomplete surgery. The extent of lymph node resection is controversial. Some advocate removal of enlarged nodes only (particularly for follicular cancers and for papillary cancers if radioiodine ablation is planned) and others central compartment removal. Radioiodine ablation is recommended after surgery to destroy remnant thyroid tissue and to facilitate surveillance with thyroglobulin assays. It is recommended for widespread local and metastatic disease (stages 3 and 4 of AJCC) and in selected patients with local disease (all patients younger than 45 years and most patients older than 45 years with stage 2 disease and patients with stage 1 disease if associated with multifocal involvement, nodal metastases, local extrathyroidal or vascular invasion and more aggressive histological types). There is good evidence from retrospective studies that shows a reduction of disease recurrence and cause-specific mortality after radioiodine ablation. Such benefit is not convincing in patients with papillary tumours with the lowest risk of mortality. Suppressive T_4 therapy, RAI uptake scans (with or without recombinant TSH) and follow-up thyroglobulin assays are done according to current protocols.

DRUGS AND THE THYROID

Drugs affect thyroid function by several mechanisms (see Table 3.7).

Amiodarone

Amiodarone contains 37% iodine by weight and causes thyroid dysfunction in up to 15% of those treated in the USA and UK. The incidence and type of dysfunction depend on the environmental iodine status; in general, hypothyroidism (amiodarone-induced hypothyroidism) is more common in iodine-sufficient areas and thyrotoxicosis (amiodarone-induced thyrotoxicosis) in iodine-deficient areas.

Table 3.7: Drugs causing thyroid dysfunction

Drug(s)	Mechanism
Dopamine, dobutamine	Inhibit TSH secretion
Glucocorticoids	Inhibit TSH secretion, thyroid hormone synthesis and release, and T_4 to T_3 deiodination
Amiodarone	Iodine-induced modification of hormone synthesis and release, inhibits T_4 to T_3 deiodination, modifies hormone action
Lithium	Inhibits hormone synthesis and release
Interleukins, interferon-α, monoclonal antibodies	Immune function modification
Beta blockers	Inhibit T_4 to T_3 deiodination
Cholecystographic agents	T_4 displacement from tissues, iodine-induced modification of thyroid hormone synthesis and release
Ipodate, iopanoic acid	Inhibit T_4 to T_3 deiodination
Heparin, aspirin, some non-steroidal anti-inflammatory drugs	Displace thyroid hormones from binding proteins
Rifampin (rifampicin)	Increases clearance of thyroid hormones
Phenytoin, carbamazepine	Increase clearance of thyroid hormones, displace hormones from binding proteins

T_3, triiodothyronine; T_4, thyroxine; TSH, thyroid-stimulating hormone.

Amiodarone inhibits deiodination of T_4 and initially causes high normal free T_4, low normal free T_3 and raised TSH level (which rapidly returns to normal).

Amiodarone-induced hypothyroidism

Very few patients with amiodarone-induced hypothyroidism are symptomatic. Moderately raised TSH (up to 20 mU/L) levels associated with high normal or raised free T_4 indicate subclinical hypothyroidism, and those with thyroid peroxidase antibodies may benefit from T_4 therapy (as most progress to permanent hypothyroidism). Higher TSH levels and low normal free T_4 indicate significant hypothyroidism and the need for treatment.

Amiodarone-induced thyrotoxicosis

There are two forms of amiodarone-induced thyrotoxicosis:

1. amiodarone-induced thyrotoxicosis type 1, due to iodine toxicity in patients with underlying thyroid disease
2. amiodarone-induced thyrotoxicosis type 2, due to a direct toxic effect of amiodarone causing a destructive thyroiditis (Table 3.8).

This subdivision is useful, as the management of amiodarone-induced thyrotoxicosis is influenced by its type, but the distinction is not always easy in clinical practice and the

Table 3.8: Amiodarone-induced thyrotoxicosis[a]

	Amiodarone-induced thyrotoxicosis type 1	Amiodarone-induced thyrotoxicosis type 2
Thyroid	Multinodular goitre or smooth goitre	Normal
Ultrasound scan	Multinodular goitre or diffuse enlargement	Normal
Colour flow Doppler scan	Normal or increased flow	Decreased flow
Thyroid antibodies	Absent or present	Absent generally
Interleukin-6	Normal or high	Very high
Radioactive iodine uptake	Low, normal or high	Very low
Preferred treatment	Carbimazole/propylthiouracil, potassium perchlorate	Glucocorticoids

[a]Amiodarone-induced thyrotoxicosis is more common in iodine-deficient areas (12%) versus iodine-sufficient areas (2%). Amiodarone-induced thyrotoxicosis type 1 is due to excess iodine (Jod–Basedow effect), and type 2 is a destructive thyroiditis. Amiodarone-induced hypothyroidism is more common in iodine-sufficient areas (13%) versus iodine-deficient areas (6%). It is caused by a decrease in thyroid hormone synthesis (inhibition of thyroidal organic iodine uptake due to an acute increase in iodide provided by amiodarone ingestion, the Wolff–Chaikoff effect), particularly in thyroid peroxidase antibody-positive patients.

two forms may coexist. Typical adrenergic features of thyrotoxicosis may be absent, but new or recurrent tachydysrhythmias or heart failure in amiodarone-treated patients should arouse suspicion of amiodarone-induced thyrotoxicosis. High or high normal free T_4, normal free T_3 and undetectable or significantly low TSH indicate only subclinical thyrotoxicosis. However, raised free T_3 levels and the above TSH abnormalities confirm amiodarone-induced thyrotoxicosis.

Management

There are inadequate data for the recommendation of routine withdrawal of amiodarone (although the indications for it should be reviewed). Amiodarone protects from the adrenergic effects of thyrotoxicosis, and withdrawal may destabilize cardiac status. Furthermore, benefits of withdrawal are not immediate. Combinations of antithyroid drugs and corticosteroids may have to be used in some patients with mixed forms of amiodarone-induced thyrotoxicosis or when tests are inconclusive. Some clinicians start with a combination and withdraw one drug depending on progress within the first few weeks. High-dose thionamide therapy is usually given for 6–12 weeks and gradual withdrawal attempted. Some need indefinite treatment. The use of perchlorate is limited by serious side-effects. RAI ablative therapy may be indicated for recurrence of amiodarone-induced thyrotoxicosis type 1 (after RAI uptake is established). Life-threatening amiodarone-induced thyrotoxicosis not responding to medical therapy may require surgery.

Interferon-α

Between 1 and 35% of patients on interferon-α manifest thyroid dysfunction caused by immune modulation and inhibition of hormone synthesis, release and metabolism. An increased risk of thyroid dysfunction occurs in female patients, in the presence of thyroid peroxidase antibodies and by the use of lymphoblastoid interferon-α. Several types of thyroid dysfunction may occur. Destructive thyroiditis produces a transient and mild thyrotoxicosis (with negative thyrotrophin receptor antibody, low RAI uptake and reduced flow on colour flow Doppler scan) in the first weeks and may lead to late hypothyroidism. Beta blockers may be required for symptom relief. Exacerbations of Graves' disease may also occur (they are thyrotrophin receptor antibody-positive and have an increased RAI uptake), requiring antithyroid drugs or RAI therapy. Hypothyroidism requiring T_4 (especially in those on combination therapy with ribavirin) occurs in 2–19% and more commonly in those with previous autoimmunity. Thyroid disease progresses in some even when interferon-α is stopped.

Lithium

About 5% of patients taking lithium develop hypothyroidism associated with thyroid autoantibodies and goitre and benefit from T_4 therapy.

RESISTANCE TO THYROID HORMONES

Thyroid hormone β-receptor mutations are largely responsible for this mainly dominantly inherited (a 'dominant negative' effect) disorder. Its incidence is estimated at one per 50 000 live births. Resistance to thyroid hormones (RTH) presents as generalized RTH or pituitary/central RTH. In both, there is RTH at the level of the pituitary or hypothalamus, with peripheral tissue resistance in addition in generalized RTH. Clinically, the majority of patients are asymptomatic, but some patients may present with goitre and signs of hypo- or euthyroidism (generalized RTH) or thyrotoxicosis (pituitary/ central RTH). A high incidence of learning and speech disabilities may also occur. Both generalized and pituitary/central RTH patients have elevated free T_4 and free T_3, with inappropriately normal (85%) or elevated TSH levels. Differential diagnosis is mainly from a TSH-secreting pituitary adenoma (Table 3.9).

There is no specific therapy for RTH. Thyroid hormone treatment is needed in patients with limited thyroid reserve (those with concomitant autoimmune thyroid disease and who have had inappropriate ablative therapy). High doses may be required, and careful monitoring is necessary. In those with hyperthyroid symptoms, symptomatic treatment with atenolol is helpful. However, triiodothyroacetic acid and D-T_4 have been used to reduce TSH and thyroid hormone levels and reduce goitre size.

THYROID DYSGENESIS

Screening for congenital hypothyroidism has helped in elucidating its causes and preventing its long-term sequelae. It is estimated that 80–85% of those with congenital hypothyroidism have thyroid dysgenesis (abnormal thyroid gland development) and 10–

Table 3.9: Differential diagnosis between thyroid-stimulating hormone-secreting pituitary adenoma and resistance to thyroid hormone

	TSH-secreting adenoma	Resistance to thyroid hormone
Family history	No	Yes
Elevated α subunit	+	–
Elevated α subunit/TSH molar ratio	+	–
Elevated sex hormone-binding globulin level	+	–
Magnetic resonance imaging scan of pituitary	Macroadenoma usually	Normal
Thyrotrophin-releasing hormone test	Impaired or absent	Normal or exaggerated
Triiodothyronine suppression test	No suppression of TSH	TSH may be suppressed
Thyroid hormone β-receptor mutation	–	+

TSH, thyroid-stimulating hormone.

15% have dyshormonogenesis. In subjects with thyroid dysgenesis, complete agenesis or hypoplasia may be associated with migration defects of the thyroid gland. Genetic defects of the transcription factors controlling organogenesis and migration, such as NKX2.1, FOXE-1 and PAX-8, account for a small minority of these patients. Loss of function mutations in the TSHR gene have also been described. There is a significant increase in associated malformations such as cardiac defects. A rare cause of severe mental retardation and neurological dysfunction (Allan–Herndon–Dudley syndrome), an X-linked disease in young males, has been found to be due to a thyroid hormone transporter (MCT8) gene mutation.

Further reading

American Thyroid Association Guidelines Taskforce 2006 Management guidelines for patients with thyroid nodules and differentiated thyroid cancer. Thyroid 16: 1–33

Braverman LE (ed.) 2003 Contemporary endocrinology: diseases of the thyroid. Humana Press, New Jersey

Braverman LE, Utiger RD (eds) 2005 Werner and Ingbar's thyroid: a fundamental and clinical text, 9th edn. Lippincott Williams & Wilkins, Philadelphia

British Thyroid Association and Royal College of Physicians 2002 Guidelines for the management of thyroid cancer in adults. BTA and RCP, London

Cooper DS 2005 Drug therapy: anti-thyroid drugs. New Engl J Med 352: 905–917

De Groot LJ, Hennemann G (eds) Thyroid disease manager. Online. Available: http://www.thyroidmanager.org

Grozinsky-Glasberg S, Fraser A, Nahshoni E et al. 2006 Thyroxine–triiodothyronine combination therapy versus thyroxine monotherapy for clinical hypothyroidism: meta-analysis of randomized controlled trials. J Clin Endocrinol Metab 91: 2592–2599

The Royal College of Physicians 2007 The use of radioiodine in the management of benign thyroid disease – clinical guidelines. RCP, London

Wass J, Shalet S (eds) 2002 Oxford textbook of endocrinology and diabetes. Oxford University Press, Oxford

Weetman A 2000 Medical progress: Graves' disease. New Engl J Med 343: 1236–1248

SELF-ASSESSMENT

Patient 1

A 34-year-old woman who takes no medication presents with increasing tiredness, weight loss of 1 stone in 2 months and a recent onset of grittiness in her eyes. She had been treated for Graves' disease with a block and replacement regimen 2 years previously. She married recently, lives with her husband and gave up her job to start a family. She smokes 20 cigarettes per day. Her mother has a goitre and takes T_4. Clinical examination reveals an anxious woman with tremors, moist palms and a pulse rate of 94 per min. There is a smooth non-tender goitre with an audible bruit, mild bilateral exophthalmos and mild swelling of the eyelids. There is no chemosis, corneal abnormalities or obvious eye muscle involvement, and her fundi are normal. Her free T_4 is 44 pmol/L (9–23 pmol/L), her TSH is less than 0.01 mU/L (0.05–4.5 mU/L) and she is positive for thyrotrophin receptor antibodies.

Questions
1. How would you manage this patient's thyrotoxicosis?
2. Would you recommend radioiodine therapy?
3. How would you counsel her?

Answers
1. This young woman has had a relapse of Graves' disease and now needs definitive therapy. However, she has prominent thyrotoxic symptoms, and propranolol 40–80 mg t.d.s. should be given to counteract the adrenergic effects of her disease (tachycardia, tremors and sweating). She should also be treated with carbimazole 40 mg daily or propylthiouracil 150 mg t.d.s., in gradually reducing doses, while she awaits definitive therapy.
2. Radioiodine therapy is effective and safe for definitive therapy of Graves' disease when adequate precautions are observed. The patient's Graves-related eye disease is non-sight-threatening as described and does not contraindicate its use. However, if doubt exists, protection would be provided by prednisolone given at a dose of 30–40 mg/day for 1 month after radioiodine therapy and gradually reduced. Pregnancy should be excluded before radioiodine therapy is given (if necessary, using a pregnancy test).
3. The patient should be counselled about the following.
   —Smoking cessation. Smoking may worsen eye disease and may have precipitated this recurrence.
   —Thionamide toxicity. The patient should be warned to look out for symptoms of fever and severe sore throat, heralding agranulocytosis. Urgent medical attention should be sought. It is wise to document such advice in the case notes.
   —Stopping thionamide therapy. She should stop thionamide drugs 3–4 days before radioiodine therapy and for 2–3 days after to maximize uptake.
   —Avoiding pregnancy. She should avoid becoming pregnant for 6–12 months (see text) to minimize potential fetal damage.

—Contact with children and vulnerable adults. The patient should avoid intimate contact with these groups for a variable period after radioiodine therapy, depending on the dose administered.

—Risk of hypothyroidism. She should be warned of the risk of long-term hypothyroidism after radioiodine therapy (see text).

—Setting off alarms. She should carry her radiation certificate, as some sensitive airport alarms may be activated, leading to unnecessary inconvenience.

—Risk of cancer. There is no increased risk of cancer following radioiodine therapy.

Patient 2

A 68-year-old retired teacher with coronary heart disease presents with palpitations that he describes as fast and irregular. His previously stable angina now occurs more frequently. He developed ventricular tachycardia after myocardial infarction several years ago. He was investigated for a 'thyroid problem' in the past. He currently takes aspirin 75 mg/day, amiodarone 200 mg/day, ramipril 10 mg/day and atorvastatin 40 mg/day. Both his parents had ischaemic heart disease, but his four adult children are healthy. He lives with his wife and is a teetotaller. On clinical examination, he is thin and has tremors and an irregular pulse of about 90 per min. He has a small smooth goitre and greyish pigmentation of his face. Free T_4 is 25 pmol/L (9–23 pmol/L), free T_3 10 pmol/L (3–5 pmol/L) and TSH less than 0.01 mU/L (0.05–4.5 mU/L). An electrocardiogram confirms atrial fibrillation.

Questions
1. What is the diagnosis and how would you investigate this patient?
2. How would you treat him?

Answers
1. This man has developed atrial fibrillation complicating clinical and biochemical thyrotoxicosis. The differential diagnosis is between Graves' disease and amiodarone-induced thyrotoxicosis. He is, however, thyrotrophin receptor antibody-negative, which excludes Graves' disease. A new onset of atrial fibrillation (or other tachydysrhythmia) or heart failure in a previously stable patient on amiodarone therapy frequently heralds the onset of amiodarone-induced thyrotoxicosis. The patient is likely to have amiodarone-induced thyrotoxicosis type 1, as he has evidence of previous thyroid disease (investigated for thyroid dysfunction) and a goitre. If available, an RAI uptake scan would show low or normal uptake (absent to very low in amiodarone-induced thyrotoxicosis type 2), and a colour flow Doppler scan would show increased flow (decreased in amiodarone-induced thyrotoxicosis type 2).
2. Carbimazole 40 mg daily (or propylthiouracil in suitable doses) should be started for control of the patient's thyrotoxicosis. Some clinicians would combine this with prednisolone 40 mg/day from the beginning (and withdraw one medication as the type of amiodarone-induced thyrotoxicosis becomes clear) or add prednisolone later if control is poor. Some patients may require combined therapy, as amiodarone-induced thyrotoxicosis type 1 and type 2 disease may occur together. Withdrawal should be

attempted in a few months, but indefinite thionamide therapy, RAI therapy or surgery may be indicated, depending on response.

Amiodarone would need to be continued in this man in view of a significant initial indication. In addition, the cardioprotective effects of amiodarone may confer benefit, and some would recommend continuation of therapy for this reason.

The patient should receive anticoagulation if no contraindications are present, as it is thought that the thromboembolic risk of thyrotoxic atrial fibrillation is high.

Disorders of calcium metabolism

M. D. Page

PHYSIOLOGY

Normal calcium balance is central to all normal cellular activity, cell signalling mechanisms and neuromuscular activity. Therefore extracellular fluid calcium levels are tightly regulated, and small perturbations can have major clinical effects. The major hormones and organs involved in calcium homeostasis are parathyroid hormone (PTH), vitamin D, the kidney, the intestine and the skeleton. Calcitonin has little or no role and will not be discussed here.

The average diet contains around 1 g of calcium per day, of which only 400–500 mg is absorbed. Some 300 mg is lost from intestinal secretions, giving a net absorption of just 100–200 mg/day. A similar amount must be lost by urinary excretion to maintain steady state. Most body calcium and phosphate exists as skeletal hydroxyapatite. In plasma, 40% of calcium is bound to albumin and 15% exists as calcium citrate or sulphate. The remaining 45% is ionized and represents the only fraction of the total under hormonal control.

Parathyroid hormone is an 84-amino acid polypeptide. Low plasma ionized calcium stimulates the calcium-sensing receptor in the cell membrane of parathyroid cells, which then release PTH. PTH raises plasma calcium by a number of linked mechanisms.

- In bone, PTH stimulates osteoclastic bone resorption with release of calcium and phosphate; vitamin D is an essential permissive agent for this action.
- In the kidney, PTH stimulates the activation of vitamin D through its actions on 1-α-hydroxylase, which then enhances intestinal calcium phosphate absorption.
- In the renal tubules, acting via cyclic AMP, PTH causes calcium resorption and phosphaturia.

Overall, in the presence of normal renal function the outcome of PTH secretion is elevation of calcium and lowering of phosphate.

Cholecalciferol (vitamin D) is a fat-soluble steroid absorbed from the diet but also synthesized in the skin from 7-dehydrocholesterol in the presence of ultraviolet light. It is hydroxylated to calcidiol in the liver by the unregulated enzyme 25-hydroxylase, and circulates bound to a specific protein. Full activation to 1,25-dihydroxy vitamin D_3 (calcitriol) is by the enzyme 1-α-hydroxylase, present in the kidney (and also in activated macrophages and T lymphocytes; see below). Activity of this enzyme is increased by PTH, hypophosphataemia and hypocalcaemia. The abilities of calcium and phosphate to regulate the production of activated vitamin D help optimize the regulatory system. Calcitriol is degraded to 24,25-dihydroxy vitamin D in the kidney by the enzyme 24-hydroxylase. This enzyme is stimulated by calcitriol itself and inhibited by PTH, both of which are appropriate regulatory actions. The main action of vitamin D is to ensure a supply of calcium and phosphate for new bone formation and to prevent symptomatic hypocalcaemia. Thus it is permissive in the PTH-induced resorption of bone and it promotes both intestinal calcium phosphate absorption and renal calcium resorption. Finally, calcitriol appropriately inhibits PTH secretion from the parathyroid.

Hypocalcaemia results in increases in PTH and calcitriol, both of which act to raise calcium, with varying effects on plasma phosphate (bone and intestinal resorption but phosphaturia). Hypophosphataemia, however, results in vitamin D activation alone, which itself reduces PTH secretion and thereby reduces bone resorption and phosphaturia. Plasma phosphate therefore rises with little or no effect on plasma calcium.

The skeleton is a dynamic system in constant flux, but normally resorption is matched by formation and total bone mass does not change. Most pathological processes affecting bone involve excessive destruction over synthesis (e.g. hyperparathyroidism, thyrotoxicosis and gonadal hormone deficiency). Osteoblasts synthesize a number of proteins, including type 1 collagen and osteocalcin, which combine to form osteoid. Osteoblasts contain alkaline phosphatase, and circulating levels of this enzyme and osteocalcin mirror overall osteogenesis. Osteoclasts are multinucleated cells, stimulated by PTH, that attach to bone surfaces, releasing acid and hydrolytic enzymes. These dissolve bone, forming a resorptive lacuna. Bone resorption releases minerals and collagen fragments including pyridinium, deoxypyridinium and the cross-linked fragments deoxypyridinoline, N-terminal collagen cross-links and C-terminal collagen cross-links.

There are a variety of specific immunoassays for markers of bone turnover. Acid and alkaline phosphatase levels reflect activity of osteoclasts and osteoblasts, respectively, and osteocalcin is a good indicator of overall osteogenesis. Urinary calcium and hydroxyproline are markers of bone resorption but are affected by dietary intake. Urinary excretion of the collagen cross-links deoxypyridinoline, N-terminal collagen cross-links and C-terminal collagen cross-links are virtually specific for type 1 collagen and therefore accurately reflect bone resorption.

OSTEOMALACIA

Osteomalacia is due to defective mineralization of osteoid and is characterized by diffuse bone tenderness, pain worsened by exercise and proximal muscle weakness. It may be suspected radiologically by the presence of pseudofractures (Looser zones; Fig. 4.1) and fractures of the ribs, vertebrae and long bones. It has a variety of causes (see Table 4.1).

Definitive diagnosis requires bone biopsy, but this is rarely required as laboratory and radiological features are usually sufficient for diagnosis and differentiation from other causes of metabolic bone disease (Table 4.2).

Vitamin D deficiency and malabsorption (and rarely resistance) are the commonest reasons for the development of osteomalacia. Vitamin D is absorbed in sufficient quantities for health from a normal balanced diet or can be synthesized in the skin. Deficiency can occur due to increased requirement, as in pregnancy and breast feeding, poor diet and/or poor sun exposure (e.g. in elderly institutionalized patients, strict vegetarians and some migrant populations). Biochemical changes include elevated alkaline phosphatase and hypocalcaemia, but definitive diagnosis requires measurement of 25-hydroxy vitamin D levels. Although a wide normal range is often quoted, from 8 to 50 ng/mL, recent guidelines indicate that a level of >30 ng/mL is necessary to prevent and treat vitamin D-deficient states. In groups at risk, notably elderly housebound persons, deficiency can be prevented either by oral administration of a daily dose of 10 μg of vitamin D or ensuring 30–60 min of sun exposure per day.

Hypophosphataemia is an important alternative cause of osteomalacia and is most commonly due to primary tubular defects causing hereditary hypophosphataemic rickets (and osteomalacia), of which the X-linked form is the most frequent. Acquired severe hypophosphataemia and osteomalacia with normal calcium metabolism should prompt a search for a mesenchymal tumour causing 'oncogenous osteomalacia', now known to be due to secretion by the tumour of the phosphaturic growth factor fibroblast growth factor-23 or phosphatonin. Whole-body technetium-99m sestamibi scanning and

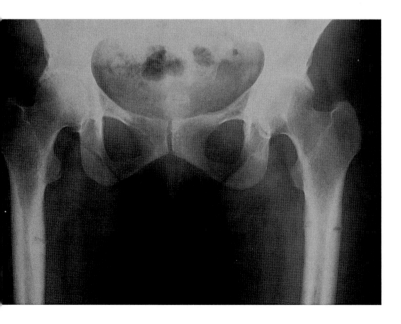

Figure 4.1
Osteomalacia. Radiograph showing Looser zones, ribbon-like demineralization in the upper femoral shaft (also found in pelvic rami, humerus, ribs and scapulae).

Table 4.1: Aetiology and treatment of osteomalacia

Mechanism	Causes	Treatment

Vitamin D deficiency
  Malnutrition
  Malabsorption
	Dietary, inadequate sunlight
	Gastrectomy, small bowel disease, pancreatic failure
		Vitamin D

Defective 25-hydroxylation	Biliary cirrhosis, alcoholic cirrhosis, drugs (e.g. anticonvulsants)	25-Hydroxy vitamin D
Defective 1-α-25-hydroxylation	Hypoparathyroidism, renal failure	1-Hydroxy vitamin D
Vitamin D resistance	Vitamin D receptor anomalies	High-dose calcitriol plus calcium
Mineralization defects	Abnormal matrix: renal failure, osteogenesis imperfecta Enzyme deficiency: hypophosphatasia Inhibitors: fluoride, aluminium, bisphosphonates	Treatment of underlying defect when possible

Phosphate deficiency	Decreased intake, antacids
	Impaired renal reabsorption
	  Primary
	  • X-linked (vitamin D-resistant)
	  • Autosomal dominant
	  • Hypophosphataemia with hypercalciuria
	  • Proximal tubular disease (Fanconi syndrome)
	  Acquired
	  • Hyperparathyroidism, primary or secondary
	  • Acquired tubular disease (myeloma)
	  • Oncogenous
		Oral phosphate and calcitriol
		
		Oral phosphate and calcitriol
		Myeloma treatment
		Tumour resection, octreotide

somatostatin scintigraphy have been shown to be an effective way of identifying these tumours, which can be very small and otherwise difficult to locate. The physiological role of phosphatonins is the subject of active investigation, as they have also been implicated in the pathogenesis of autosomal dominant hypophosphataemic rickets.

Treatment of osteomalacia involves identifying and reversing the underlying pathology, correction of hypocalcaemia and hypophosphataemia, and amelioration of any secondary hyperparathyroidism. Vitamin D itself is cheap but takes several weeks to become effective, and the biochemical effect persists for weeks after discontinuation. Various analogues, hydroxylated at the 1 (α-calcidol), 25 (calcidiol) or both (calcitriol) positions, are available and are used for specific indications (Table 4.1). In all situations, the commonest problem with treatment is the development of hypercalcaemia and hypercalciuria, leading to nephrocalcinosis and ocular calcium deposits. Hence, patients must be closely monitored as long as treatment continues.

Table 4.2: Investigations in bone disease

Condition	Calcium	Phosphate	Alkaline phosphatase	Parathyroid hormone	25-Hydroxy vitamin D	1,25-Dihydroxy vitamin D_3	Urinary calcium	Others
Vitamin D-deficient osteomalacia	Normal or ↓	Normal or ↓	↑	↑	↓	Normal or ↓	↓	–
Tubular phosphate wasting	Normal	↓	Normal	Normal	Normal	Normal	Normal	Hypouricaemia, aminoaciduria, glycosuria suggest Fanconi syndrome
Hypophosphatasia	Normal	Normal	↓	Normal	Normal	Normal	Normal	–
Primary hyper-parathyroidism	↑	↓	Normal or ↑	↑	Normal	↓	↑	–
Osteoporosis	Normal	Normal	Normal	Normal	Normal	Normal	Normal	–

Primary hypophosphataemic conditions require oral phosphate, with or without additional vitamin D analogues, to minimize secondary hyperparathyroidism. This can be very difficult to treat, because the efficacy of phosphate therapy may be limited by the dose frequency required and by troublesome side-effects including nausea and diarrhoea.

RENAL OSTEODYSTROPHY

Bone disease in renal failure can be severe and debilitating. Although rarely clinically apparent until a patient is on renal replacement therapy, the pathological process begins with falls of glomerular filtration rate (GFR) to 50 mL/min or below and needs to be considered in all patients with earlier stages of nephropathy. Patients may experience bone pain, fractures, metastatic calcification and calciphylaxis – an intensely painful necrotic ulceration of the trunk and extremities caused by arterial calcification. Phosphate retention due to tubular dysfunction begins with a GFR of <50 mL/min, before any rise is seen in creatinine. Hyperphosphataemia induces PTH secretion and also reduces the activation of 25-hydroxy vitamin D. This effect, plus falling renal mass, results in low calcitriol levels with GFR <30 mL/min. Hypocalcaemia then develops, with corresponding worsening of hyperparathyroidism. Although this is an appropriate response and in the early stages actually serves to lower phosphate levels, it contributes to the worsening of bone disease. Ultimately, autonomous parathyroid adenomas can develop, leading to tertiary hyperparathyroidism and hypercalcaemia.

Three distinct bone diseases can complicate renal failure and may coexist. Osteoporosis and osteitis fibrosa cystica can complicate hyperparathyroidism in renal failure. Osteomalacia results from failure of calcitriol production. It was previously also induced by use of aluminium-containing phosphate binders. Adynamic bone disease is increasingly common in dialysis patients. In this condition, there is reduced bone turnover but no increase in osteoid. It is not fully understood but may be related to excessive suppression of PTH by modern treatment regimens and possibly the use of calcium carbonate and calcitriol.

Management of renal osteodystrophy involves repeated measurement of calcium, phosphate and PTH, more frequently with advancing renal failure. The renal services national service framework has indicated treatment targets for the following.

- Phosphate: 1.2–1.7 mmol/L
- Calcium: within normal laboratory range
- PTH: two to three times local normal range.

25-Hydroxy vitamin D levels are required in those who develop hyperparathyroidism in order to direct therapy. Table 4.3 gives treatment recommendations. All patients with fractures and/or osteoporosis risk should have dual energy x-ray absorptiometry (DEXA) scanning, but plain radiology and bone biopsy are rarely required – even in those with end-stage renal failure.

Table 4.3: Treatment of renal bone disease

	Details
Hyperphosphataemia	
Target	1.2–1.7 mmol/L
First line	Dietary restriction ± calcium-containing binders
Resistant cases	Sevelamer ± combination of binders
Calcium >2.55 mmol/L or parathyroid hormone less than twice normal Metastatic or vascular calcification	Avoid calcium-containing binders; restrict total daily calcium intake (binders plus diet) to <2000 mg
Hypocalcaemia and hyperparathyroidism	
Hypocalcaemia target	Within laboratory normal range
Hyperparathyroidism target	Two to three times normal range
Calcium < 2.1 mmol/L ± increased parathyroid hormone	Calcium carbonate ± 1-hydroxy vitamin D
25-Hydroxy vitamin D < 30 ng/mL	Ergocalciferol

OSTEOPOROSIS

With more people surviving into their eighties and nineties, osteoporosis has become one of the most important public health problems facing the UK National Health Service today. The incidence of hip fracture rises exponentially from the age of 44 in women (after the menopause) and 75 in men, with rates over the age of 85 of $300/10^5$ for men and $500/10^5$ for women. Vertebral and wrist fractures are the other sites typically affected.

Osteoporosis is characterized by reduced bone mass and disruption of microarchitecture. There is thinning of cortical and trabecular bone due to progressive resorption until cross-bridging is lost and individual spicules of trabecular bone no longer support one another, contributing to reduced mechanical strength (Fig. 4.2). Many conditions are associated with osteoporosis (Table 4.4), but the majority of cases are age-related or postmenopausal.

In osteoporosis, low-impact fractures occur in typical sites (Fig. 4.3) and the trauma may be so minor as to be unrecalled, especially for vertebral fractures. Therefore osteoporosis is a silent condition until a fracture occurs. This is an important practice point, as patients often assume wrongly that their bone pain is due to osteoporosis. Pain without fracture should prompt a search for alternative pathology, including arthritis, osteomalacia, Paget's disease or malignancy.

The assessment required for osteoporosis is shown in Table 4.5. DEXA scanning provides a reliable measure of bone mineral density (BMD). X-rays of dual energy are produced by the tube and quantified after passing through the patient. The different energy rays are variably attenuated by bone, allowing integration of data to provide a measurement of

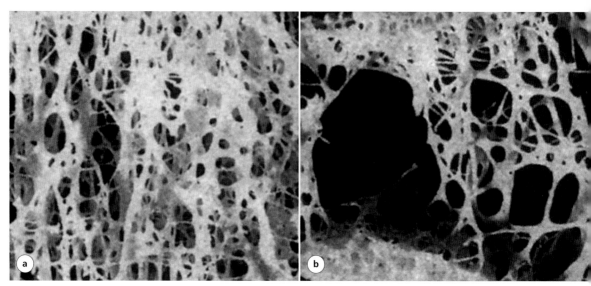

Figure 4.2
(a) Normal and (b) osteoporotic bone. Note the thinning of trabeculae and disruption of architecture, resulting in reduced mechanical strength.

Table 4.4: Aetiology of osteoporosis

	Details
Common	Postmenopausal Age-related Familial
Endocrine and metabolic	Hypogonadism (all causes) Glucocorticoid excess (endogenous or therapeutic) Hyperthyroidism (includes 'subclinical' and over-replacement with thyroxine) Hyperparathyroidism Growth hormone or insulin-like growth factor-1 deficiency Homocystinuria
Malnutrition	Vitamin D deficiency Low calcium intake Malabsorption Coeliac disease Cystic fibrosis Anorexia nervosa
Drugs	Glucocorticoids Heparin (long-term use, e.g. in pregnancy) Cyclosporin Medroxyprogesterone (e.g. Depo-Provera) Vitamin A Anticonvulsants
Systemic disease	Liver disease Rheumatic disease (rheumatoid arthritis, systemic lupus erythematosus)
Miscellaneous	Smoking Alcohol Inactive lifestyle

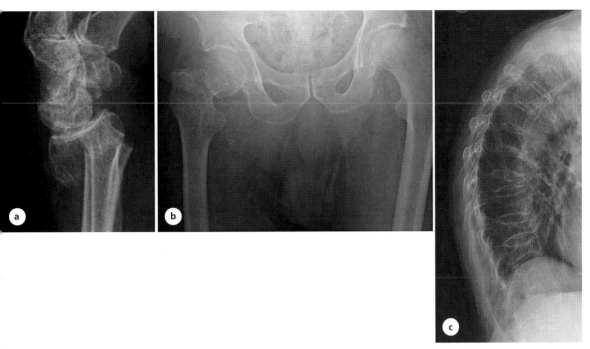

Figure 4.3

Osteoporotic fractures: **(a)** Colles wrist fracture, **(b)** subcapital fracture (right hip), **(c)** multiple vertebral body fractures with kyphosis and loss of height.

Table 4.5: Diagnosis and assessment of osteoporosis

Clinical feature(s)	Investigations
Vertebral fracture (60% without symptoms): • usually D7–12 • back pain • kyphosis, pain from neck hyperextension • loss of height, protuberant abdomen • pain from ribs and iliac crests	Measurement of bone density • X-rays: typical fractures and vertebral morphology; unreliable for demonstration of 'osteopenia' • Dual energy x-ray absorptiometry: investigation of choice; high precision and intraindividual reproducibility; lateral scanning reduces interference from osteophytes • Qualitative computerized tomography: research tool
Hip and wrist fractures: low impact but rare without some trauma	Bone biopsy provides definitive evidence but rarely required
Miscellaneous: pathologies associated with osteoporosis	Laboratory investigation (to exclude other pathologies): full blood count, erythrocyte sedimentation rate/viscosity, urea and electrolytes and bicarbonate, liver function tests, immunoglobulins and Bence Jones protein, calcium, thyroxine/thyroid-stimulating hormone, testosterone in men; other investigations only if clinically indicated

BMD. The radiation dose is <10% that of a single chest film. Most scanners permit lateral as well as anteroposterior lumbar spine imaging, which may be important when a patient has significant degenerative arthritis with osteophyte formation. DEXA results are interpreted according to BMD as a T score, giving the standard deviation score relative to mean peak bone mass in young adults, and the Z score relative to age-matched controls; however, the Z score is not relevant to therapeutic choices and should be ignored. The clinical classification of osteoporosis is as shown in Table 4.6.

Treatment and prevention of osteoporosis

Treatment strategies are summarized in Table 4.7. Patients identified with osteopenia or osteoporosis need to have confounding problems eliminated or minimized.

Table 4.6: Clinical classification of osteoporosis

Normal bone mineral density	T score
Normal	> –1 SDs
Osteopenia	–1 to –2.5 SDs
Osteoporosis	< –2.5 SDs
Severe (complicated) osteoporosis	< –2.5 SDs plus low-impact fracture

Table 4.7: Treatment of osteoporosis

Stage of osteoporosis	Intervention	Dosage
Prevention	Smoking cessation Reduce alcohol consumption Weight-bearing exercise Calcium intake >1000 mg/day	–
Therapeutic glucocorticoids	As above *plus* bisphosphonates, calcium and vitamin D	–
Hypogonadal states	Hormone replacement therapy regimens	
Osteopenia	As above *plus* calcium with vitamin D tablets	Calcichew D Forte, two daily (20 µg of vitamin D plus 1200 mg of calcium)
Osteoporosis	As above *plus*: • etidronate • alendronate • risedronate • pamidronate • zolendronate	 Cycles of 2 weeks 400 mg o.d. followed by 11 weeks of calcium 70 mg p.o. weekly 35 mg p.o. weekly 60 mg i.v. every 3 months 1–4 mg over 1 year
Complicated/resistant osteoporosis	As above *plus*: • falls assessment • parathyroid hormone • strontium ranelate	 – 20–40 µg s.c. daily 2 g p.o. daily

- Glucocorticoid doses should be as low as possible.
- Smoking and alcohol consumption should be reduced.
- Dietary calcium should be increased to a minimum of 1000 mg/day and advice given on a weight-bearing exercise programme.

Calcium plus vitamin D tablets (two daily providing 20 μg of vitamin D plus 1200 mg of calcium) are commonly used in patients with osteopenia, along with other lifestyle interventions.

Testosterone replacement is effective in osteoporotic men with hypogonadism from any cause (including the increasingly recognized case of the middle-aged or elderly man with low testosterone and no other evidence of endocrine disease). Likewise, women with osteoporosis and hypogonadism occurring before the menopause need oestrogen replacement, often conveniently given as the combined oral contraceptive pill or standard hormone replacement therapy (HRT) regimens.

In postmenopausal women, HRT reliably preserves and will often improve BMD, particularly in the axial skeleton. However, with increasing evidence of the risks of HRT and perceived lack of benefit on cardiovascular risk and mortality, HRT has become less attractive as a first-line treatment of established osteoporosis, but there is an additive effect when used in combination with bisphosphonates in severe or resistant cases.

Bisphosphonates have become the standard first-line drugs for the treatment and prevention of osteoporosis in both men and women. A large body of data now exists demonstrating the effectiveness of these agents in terms of preserved and improved BMD and reduced fracture rates. Etidronate has the longest history of clinical use and is well tolerated when used in cyclical regimens with high-dose calcium supplements, but it is difficult to use in practice and is being replaced by newer agents including alendronate and risedronate, which are given orally on a weekly basis, and pamidronate, which can be given by intravenous infusion at 3-monthly intervals. There are promising data with zolendronate, which is a once-yearly intravenous infusion. However, intravenous (and rarely oral) bisphosphonates have been associated with osteonecrosis of the jaw. Dental hygiene should therefore be optimized prior to therapy initiation with these newer agents.

Although seemingly illogical, synthetic PTH 1–34 (teriparatide) is now licensed for use in osteoporosis that is resistant to standard treatment. It has an anabolic effect, increasing BMD in both cortical and trabecular bone in men and women. Combined teriparatide and bisphosphonates have not been shown to confer additional benefit. In fact, alendronate has been shown to blunt the anabolic benefits of teriparatide, and bisphosphonates should therefore be discontinued when treatment with teriparatide is commenced.

Strontium ranelate given orally at a dose of 2 g/day has been shown to be an effective alternative treatment in those who do not respond to or who cannot take bisphosphonates. It has effects on both bone resorption and bone formation. Although BMD measured by DEXA scanning can be falsely high in patients on strontium, this drug has been shown to have an early effect to reduce fracture frequency.

Selective oestrogen receptor modulators such as raloxifene may prove more effective and safer than conventional HRT. Growth hormone and insulin-like growth factor-1 increase BMD in growth hormone-deficient patients, but their use is restricted to patients with growth hormone deficiency syndromes. Finally, it is important to stress the effectiveness of bisphosphonates and calcium with vitamin D in the prevention of glucocorticoid-induced osteoporosis. No patient should now receive pharmacological doses of steroids without being considered for primary preventive treatment of glucocorticoid-induced osteoporosis.[1]

The National Institute for Health and Clinical Excellence has recently published draft guidance on primary and secondary prevention of osteoporosis, including recommendations for the use of all the agents mentioned above. A final guideline is likely to be available early in 2007.

HYPERCALCAEMIA

The basic mechanisms of hypercalcaemia include increased resorption from bone, from the gastrointestinal tract and from the renal tubule. Box 4.1 lists the causes of

---

Box 4.1: Causes of hypercalcaemia

Bone resorption

- Primary or tertiary hyperparathyroidism
- Cancer
    Lytic metastases
    Tumour production of parathyroid hormone-related peptide
- Hyperthyroidism
- Paget's disease (fracture or immobilization)
- Hypervitaminosis A or retinoic acid

Gastrointestinal absorption

- Milk alkali syndrome
- Vitamin D-dependent
    Oral administration
    Granulomatous disease (e.g. sarcoid)
    Malignant lymphoma

Miscellaneous

- Other endocrine conditions
    Acromegaly and multiple endocrine neoplasia type 1
    Phaeochromocytoma and multiple endocrine neoplasia type 2
    Hypoadrenal crisis
- Lithium therapy
- Thiazides
- Acute renal failure, especially after rhabdomyolysis
- Theophylline toxicity
- Familial hypocalciuric hypercalcaemia
- Immobilization
- Parenteral nutrition

hypercalcaemia. The frequency of each cause depends on the population. Therefore primary hyperparathyroidism is responsible for 90% of ambulatory cases, but malignancy accounts for 50–60% of cases in hospital.

Primary hyperparathyroidism is now most commonly diagnosed fortuitously in asymptomatic patients by 'routine' biochemical testing carried out for other reasons. Investigation of renal stone disease, osteoporosis, dementia and gastrointestinal conditions discloses other cases. Hyperparathyroid bone disease (Fig. 4.4) is now very uncommon. A single adenoma is responsible for more than 95% of cases, the remainder being associated with four-gland hyperplasia. In mild disease, PTH levels may be at the high end of the normal range and the calcium may be only intermittently elevated and can be lowered by coexisting vitamin D deficiency, such that multiple measurements may be needed to make a firm diagnosis. Differentiation of these mild cases from familial hypocalciuric hypercalcaemia, in which the calcium-sensing receptor is relatively insensitive to ionized calcium, can be difficult and relies on obtaining a family history of hypercalcaemia (often with failed neck exploration) and demonstrating hypocalciuria in the presence of hypercalcaemia. In practice, this is best done using a random urine calcium measurement with adjustment for creatinine excretion. In equivocal cases, genetic testing for mutations in the calcium-sensing receptor can be extremely helpful.

In advanced renal failure, hypercalcaemia with normal or elevated PTH can complicate the use of the oral phosphate binder calcium carbonate, particularly if vitamin D analogues are also being prescribed. The alternative phosphate binder sevelamer may be substituted, but in late disease so-called tertiary hyperparathyroidism may ensue, thought to be due to adenomatous transformation of hyperplastic parathyroid tissue.

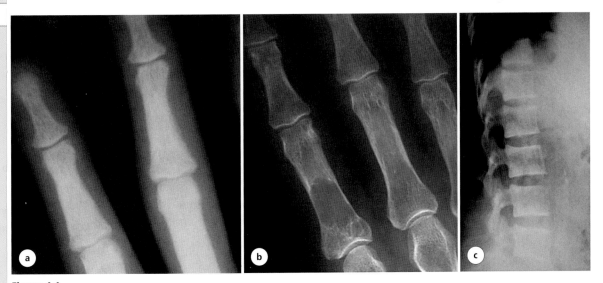

Figure 4.4
Hyperparathyroid bone disease. **(a)** Subperiosteal resorption of phalanges (common). **(b)** Brown tumour, second proximal phalanx (uncalcified osteoid), which can fracture (rare). **(c)** 'Rugger jersey spine', alternating sclerotic and lytic areas (rare).

for years, they can be destabilized by prescription of other drugs (e.g. thiazides), by dietary change and by life events (e.g. pregnancy and breast feeding).

Pseudohypoparathyroidism (PHP) describes a rare group of conditions in which there is unresponsiveness to PTH in target tissues (kidney and bone). In common with most peptide hormones, the action of PTH is mediated through a specific, membrane-associated G protein-coupled receptor. PHP usually occurs because of inactivating mutations in the Gs alpha gene (GNAS-1), leading to reduced activation of adenylate cyclase and end-organ unresponsiveness to PTH. Clinically, this is typically seen in children who are hypocalcaemic and hyperphosphataemic with secondary hyperparathyroidism. Phenotypic markers (termed *Albright's hereditary osteodystrophy*) include the following (Fig. 4.5):

- round facies
- short stature
- short third, fourth and fifth metacarpals
- obesity
- subcutaneous calcification
- developmental delay.

Hyperparathyroid bone disease will develop without treatment with vitamin D. Three forms of PHP are recognized:

1. type 1a
2. type 1b
3. pseudo-PHP.

Patients with PHP type 1a exhibit the biochemical abnormalities and Albright hereditary osteodystrophy, patients with PHP type 1b have the biochemical abnormalities alone, and patients with pseudo-PHP have Albright hereditary osteodystrophy alone without

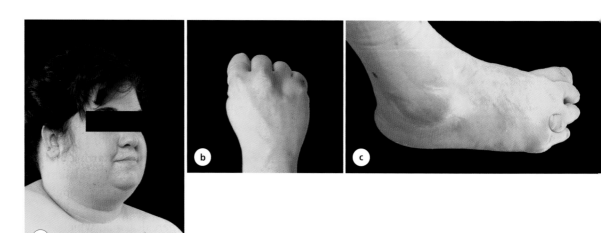

Figure 4.5
Features of pseudohypoparathyroidism.

biochemical features of PTH resistance. These differences are explained at least in part by the phenomenon of parental imprinting, by which disease expression is dependent on which parent the mutated allele is inherited from. PHP type 1a occurs only when the mutation is inherited from a mother with PHP type 1a or pseudo-PHP, whereas transmission of a mutated paternal GNAS-1 gene results in pseudo-PHP with retained calcium homeostasis due to normal maternal gene expression in the kidney. GNAS-1 is also expressed predominantly from the maternal allele in the thyroid, pituitary and gonads. Patients with PHP type 1a may therefore show evidence of resistance to thyroid-stimulating hormone, luteinizing hormone, follicle-stimulating hormone and gonadotrophin-releasing hormone, and defects in these systems should be screened for and treated appropriately. Mutations in the coding region of GNAS-1 have not been reported in PHP type 1b, which is assumed to be due to a defect in the PTH receptor.

In managing hypocalcaemia, magnesium deficiency should be actively sought and corrected by supplementation, as it can both cause hypocalcaemia via PTH suppression and impair correction of hypocalcaemia via PTH resistance. Patients with hypocalcaemia and hyperphosphataemia (e.g. tumour lysis syndrome) should receive aggressive treatment of the hyperphosphataemia as a first step (binders, dialysis), otherwise calcium can be precipitated extraskeletally.

Although PTH is a logical treatment for hypoparathyroidism and is now available for use in resistant osteoporosis, it is expensive and has to be given parenterally. It remains to be seen whether PTH will find a place in the management of the rare patient whose condition cannot be easily controlled with oral calcium salts and vitamin D analogues.

PAGET'S DISEASE OF BONE

Paget's disease is a focal disorder of the skeleton in which accelerated bone turnover with abnormal architecture results in reduced strength with deformation, liability to fracture and increased local blood flow. The aetiology is presently unknown, although it is observed that there are familial clusters suggesting either a genetic link or a viral basis. There are histological studies indicating the presence of viral particles in the osteoblasts from pagetic bone. The disease becomes progressively more common with increasing age. Autopsy and radiological studies have shown the disease to be present in over 3% after the age of 40.

Pathologically, the first event is increased osteoclastic bone resorption. Lytic fronts advance along the long bones and form circumscribed lesions in the skull (Fig. 4.6). The osteoblastic response follows, with accelerated deposition of disorganized lamellar bone. The clinical features affect a variety of organ systems and are shown in Table 4.11.

Serum calcium and phosphate are normal in most patients unless they have very active disease and after fracture with immobilization. Otherwise, hypercalcaemia suggests an alternative second pathology. Urinary excretion of hydroxyproline and pyridinoline cross-links, along with serum alkaline phosphatase and osteocalcin, is correlated with disease

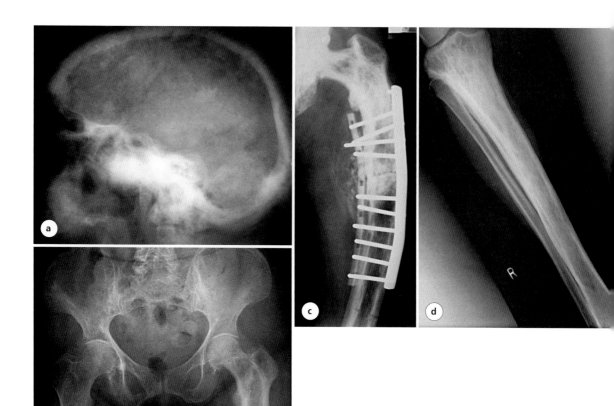

Figure 4.6
Paget's disease of bone. Affected bone shows disorganized internal structure with adjacent areas of sclerotic and lytic trabecular bone and thickened cortex. **(a)** Skull: thickened skull tables and cotton wool appearance. **(b)** Pelvis: generalized pagetic changes of pelvis and bowing of the left femur, which has a markedly thickened cortex. **(c)** Femur: there is a healing plated fracture; a second 'fissure fracture' is seen below the plate. **(d).** Tibia: thickened sclerotic bone of the upper tibia; there is a resorption front advancing into the distal tibia.

Table 4.11: Clinical features of Paget's disease

System	Feature	Details
Skeleton	Pain	Either direct from the lesion or secondary to local deformity and osteoarthritis
	Deformity	Thickened and bowed long bones, mechanical stress, enlargement of the skull
	Fracture	Traumatic or pathological, often incomplete, healing usually normal
	Tumours	Increased osteosarcoma risk
Neurological	Nerve compression	Eighth nerve, other cranial nerves, spinal nerve roots
	Basal skull invagination	Aqueduct blockage and hydrocephalus
Cardiac	Heart failure	Increased output to hypervascular bone

Table 4.12: Treatments for Paget's disease

Treatment	Details
Bisphosphonates	Pyrophosphate analogues bind to bone and render it less susceptible to osteoclastic resorption; poorly absorbed orally Pamidronate widely used, but alendronate, risedronate, tiludronate and zolendronate all effective as intermittent intravenous infusions
Calcitonin	Either subcutaneous or nasal spray; expensive and associated with nausea, flushing and allergic reactions; occasionally used in combination with bisphosphonates in resistant cases
Gallium	–

activity and extent and with response to treatment. It should be noted that normal values can be found in patients with limited, especially mono-ostotic disease. In most cases, a clinical assessment with measurement of calcium, phosphate, alkaline phosphatase and urine hydroxyproline and with plain radiography of affected areas and bone scanning is all that is necessary to determine the extent and activity of disease and to assess response to treatment.

The indications for treatment include pain from pagetic bone, headache from skull disease, hypercalcaemia after immobilization, before elective surgery on affected bones (to reduce hypervascularity) and to prevent nerve compression developing. Therefore asymptomatic patients may require prophylactic treatment. Improvement of existing neurocompressive symptoms is unlikely to occur. Pain from secondary osteoarthritis may not improve with antipagetic treatment. Corrective orthopaedic surgery is often required. The agents available for treatment are shown in Table 4.12. In effect, all successful disease-modifying treatments suppress osteoclastic activity.

References

1. Royal College of Physicians 2002 Glucocorticoid induced osteoporosis: guideline for treatment and prevention. RCP, London

Further reading

De Groot LJ, Jameson JL (eds) 2005 Endocrinology, 5th edn. Saunders, Philadelphia

Farfel Z, Bourne HR, Iiri T 1999 The expanding spectrum of G protein diseases. New Engl J Med 340: 1012–1020

Meunier PJ, Roux C, Seeman E et al. 2004 The effects of strontium ranelate on the risk of vertebral fracture in women with postmenopausal osteoporosis. New Engl J Med 350: 459–468

Rubin MR, Bilezikian JP 2005 Parathyroid hormone as an anabolic skeletal therapy. Drugs 65: 2481–2498

SELF-ASSESSMENT

Patient 1

A 45-year-old man presents with back pain. A wrist fracture sustained skiing had healed successfully 1 year earlier. Imaging shows wedge fractures of D9 and 10. The radiologist reports the fractures and comments that the bones look generally osteopenic.

Questions
1. What must be elicited from the history?
2. What investigations should be requested?

A DEXA scan shows T scores of −3.6 in the lumbar spine and −4.1 in the hip.

3. What advice would you give the patient?
4. What treatment should be considered?
5. How should he be followed up?

Answers
1. The patient should be asked about family history of fragility fractures, a history of each fracture, and symptoms and signs of endocrine disease (hypercalcaemia, hypogonadism, Cushing's syndrome, thyrotoxicosis). Drug, smoking and alcohol histories should be assessed, as should symptoms suggestive of malabsorption, coeliac disease, myeloma or malignancy.
2. Investigations should include calcium, phosphate, alkaline phosphatase, myeloma screen, blood count, and renal and liver profile. Endocrine tests required include testosterone, prolactin and thyroid function tests. Other tests should not be performed unless clinically indicated.
3. This man has severe complicated osteoporosis. Confounding conditions should be aggressively treated. He should receive advice to limit his alcohol consumption and not to smoke. Regular aerobic exercise, avoiding high-impact stress, should be recommended. He should have a good balanced diet with calcium intake supplemented to at least 2 g/day.
4. Because the patient has already lost significant bone density and is at risk of further fractures, specific therapy should be with an anabolic agent. Teriparatide is indicated for this man and should probably be his first-line therapy.
5. A follow-up DEXA scan should be carried out at 6 months to assess response to treatment, and annually thereafter.

Patient 2

A 51-year-old woman is referred for assessment of hypercalcaemia found by chance at a well woman screening clinic at her surgery. The calcium is 2.78 mmol/L and phosphate is 0.89 mmol/L. The remainder of her biochemical profile, including alkaline phosphatase, is normal.

Question
1. What do you need to know and what investigations are required?

Answer
1. The history should explore the use of calcium-elevating drugs and vitamin preparations, symptoms of renal stone disease and fractures, and family history of endocrine disease and neck operations. Investigations should include full blood count, biochemical profile, thyroid function tests, PTH, an estimation of urine calcium excretion and a chest x-ray.

The patient's PTH is returned at 7.8 pg/mL (2.5–7.5 pg/mL) and the calcium:creatinine ratio on an early morning sample is 0.8 (0.1–0.4). All other investigations are normal.

Questions
2. What is the diagnosis?
3. Are any other investigations required?
4. What treatment should be considered?

Answers
2. The patient has asymptomatic primary hyperparathyroidism. The elevated urine calcium excludes familial hypocalciuric hypercalcaemia, and there are no other conditions in which calcium is elevated in the face of unsuppressed PTH.
3. Because the treatment decision is between parathyroidectomy and observation, absolute indications for neck exploration should be sought. These would include calcium more than 2.85 mmol/L, an episode of severe hypercalcaemia, severe hypercalciuria more than 400 mg/24 h or established nephrolithiasis, impaired renal function, osteoporosis and age less than 50 years. The patient should go on to have her 24-h urine calcium excretion measured, a DEXA scan and imaging of her renal tract, looking for calcification.
4. If her additional tests do not give an absolute indication for surgery, she may be offered observation as an alternative. In the event that she elects to be observed, she should be reviewed with repeat calcium on a 6-monthly basis. Repeat DEXA scanning and 24-h urine calcium excretion should be repeated at 2-year intervals.

Adrenal disorders

J. Smith

ANATOMY AND PHYSIOLOGY

The adrenal cortex is divided into three histological and functional zones:

1. the outer, aldosterone-secreting zona glomerulosa
2. the intermediate, cortisol-secreting zona fasciculata
3. the inner, androgen-secreting zona reticularis.

Whereas the zona glomerulosa is primarily regulated by angiotensin II, both the zona fasciculata and the zona reticularis are regulated by adrenocorticotrophic hormone (ACTH). Utilizing cholesterol as a precursor molecule, the adrenal cortex is responsible for the synthesis of steroid hormones (Fig. 5.1).

Glucocorticoids are key hormones involved in cardiovascular, metabolic and immune homeostasis, and the hypothalamic–pituitary–adrenal axis plays a pivotal role in the stressor response. Cortisol exerts negative feedback control on corticotrophin-releasing hormone/vasopressin in the hypothalamus and ACTH in the pituitary. Cortisol is secreted in a circadian rhythm, with levels falling during the day from a peak at 7–8 a.m. to a nadir at around midnight.

Only a very small fraction of circulating cortisol is in the free state, with approximately 80–90% being bound to a specific globulin, cortisol-binding globulin (CBG), and approximately 5–10% bound to albumin. Because current assays measure total levels of cortisol (bound and unbound), changes in CBG induced by other hormones (e.g. oestrogen and thyroid hormones increase CBG synthesis) are important to recognize, as these may increase measured levels of cortisol without affecting biologically active free levels.

The principal mineralocorticoid, aldosterone, acts primarily at the renal distal convoluted tubule, and its synthesis is largely regulated by the renin–angiotensin system (Fig. 5.2). Renin is produced in the juxtaglomerular apparatus of the kidney and catalyses the conversion of inactive angiotensinogen to angiotensin I. This undergoes further enzymatic conversion by angiotensin-converting enzyme (ACE) to produce angiotensin II, which acts via the angiotensin receptor to stimulate the release of aldosterone. Aldosterone production is also regulated to some degree by potassium balance (low potassium inhibits secretion) and ACTH.

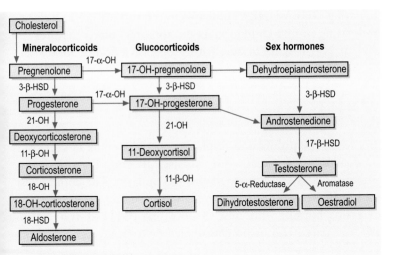

Figure 5.1
Adrenal steroid biosynthesis. HSD, hydroxysteroid dehydrogenase; OH, hydroxylase.

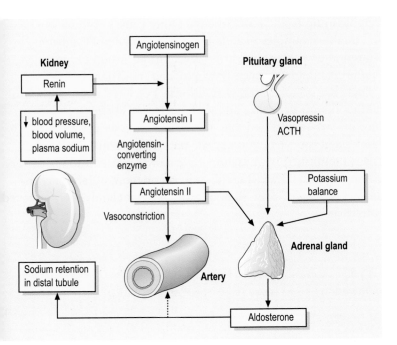

Figure 5.2
The renin–angiotensin–aldosterone system. ACTH, adrenocorticotrophic hormone.

Adrenal androgens, controlled mainly by ACTH, are steroid hormones with weak androgenic activity. They are thought to have only a relatively minor role in adult men and are more physiologically important in the adult woman and in both sexes before puberty. The major adrenal androgens are dehydroepiandrosterone (DHEA), DHEA sulphate and androstenedione, all of which may be converted to the more potent androgens testosterone and dihydrotestosterone in peripheral tissues. Major peripheral sites of androgen conversion are the hair follicles, the sebaceous glands, the prostate and the external genitalia. Circulating DHEA/DHEA sulphate concentrations are low during infancy and early childhood, rising in mid-childhood as the zona reticularis matures (*adrenarche*) to reach a peak at 20–30 years of age, with progressive decline thereafter.

ADRENAL INSUFFICIENCY

Adrenal insufficiency occurs when the production of glucocorticoids, mineralocorticoids and adrenal androgens is reduced. It can be caused by diseases affecting the adrenal cortex (primary) or the pituitary gland and hypothalamus (secondary). The commonest cause of secondary adrenal insufficiency is suppression of hypothalamic–pituitary function (corticotrophin-releasing hormone–arginine vasopressin–ACTH axis) by chronic exogenous glucocorticoids (oral, parenteral or potent inhaled or topical preparations).

The causes of primary adrenal insufficiency (Addison's disease) are shown in Box 5.1. Autoimmune adrenalitis is now the predominant cause of primary adrenal insufficiency in western populations, and antibodies directed against specific enzymes (e.g. 21-hydroxylase) may be detectable in up to 90% of patients. Other causes are rare but should not be overlooked. Notable examples include the antiphospholipid syndrome, in which bilateral adrenal infarction due to adrenal arterial/venous occlusion may precipitate acute adrenal failure, and adrenoleucodystrophy and its variant adrenomyeloneuropathy. These are X-linked recessive disorders of fatty acid metabolism that usually present in childhood with dementia and limb paralysis. However, presentations in adolescence or early adulthood may occur, and they should be considered in the differential diagnosis when young male patients present with adrenal insufficiency. The diagnosis is established by measuring circulating concentrations of very long chain fatty acids. Although adrenal metastatic disease is common, adrenal failure due to metastatic infiltration is rare, with over 90% of both adrenal glands needing to be affected before gland failure ensues.

Box 5.1: Causes of primary adrenal insufficiency

- Autoimmune (including polyglandular failure)
- Tuberculosis
- Sarcoidosis, amyloidosis, haemochromatosis
- Haemorrhage (meningococcaemia, anticoagulants, trauma)
- Bilateral infarction secondary to antiphospholipid syndrome
- Fungal infections (e.g. histoplasmosis)
- Metastatic neoplasia or infiltration
- Congenital adrenal hyperplasia
- Congenital adrenal hypoplasia
- Adrenoleucodystrophy
- AIDS
- Bilateral adrenalectomy
- Steroid synthesis inhibitors (e.g. metyrapone, ketoconazole, etomidate, aminoglutethimide)

Box 5.2: Autoimmune polyglandular syndromes

Autoimmune polyglandular syndrome type 1

- Autosomal recessive inheritance
- Hypoparathyroidism (90%)
- Primary adrenal insufficiency (60%)
- Primary hypothyroidism
- Primary gonadal failure
- Hypopituitarism (rare)

Non-endocrine associations

- Mucocutaneous candidiasis
- Pernicious anaemia
- Vitiligo
- Chronic active hepatitis
- Malabsorption

Autoimmune polyglandular syndrome type 2

- Autosomal recessive or dominant inheritance
- Primary adrenal insufficiency (100%)
- Primary hypothyroidism
- Primary gonadal failure
- Type 1 diabetes

Non-endocrine associations

- Myasthenia gravis
- Alopecia
- Pernicious anaemia
- Vitiligo
- Immune thrombocytopenic purpura

Approximately 50% of patients with autoimmune adrenal insufficiency will also have evidence of one or more other autoimmune endocrine disorders. The occurrence of autoimmune adrenal insufficiency in combination with other autoimmune endocrine and non-endocrine disorders is collectively referred to as the autoimmune polyglandular syndromes, of which there are broadly two types (1 and 2). The principal features of these are shown in Box 5.2.

Clinical features

The development of adrenal insufficiency is often gradual and may go undetected until an illness or other stress precipitates an adrenal crisis. Patients may present to a variety of different specialists because of the non-specific nature of their symptoms, and clinicians must always maintain a high index of suspicion for the diagnosis.

The most common clinical features of chronic primary adrenal insufficiency include:

- general malaise
- fatigue
- weakness
- anorexia
- weight loss

115

- nausea
- vomiting
- abdominal pain
- diarrhoea.

In addition, postural hypotension, electrolyte abnormalities (hyponatraemia, hyperkalaemia, metabolic acidosis), hyperpigmentation (due to ACTH excess from loss of cortisol negative feedback) and autoimmune manifestations (e.g. vitiligo) may also occur. Additional laboratory abnormalities include elevated urea, increased plasma renin activity, mild hypercalcaemia, and anaemia (normocytic normochromic) with eosinophilia. There may also be a reduction in thyroid hormone levels and elevated thyroid-stimulating hormone, due to either a transient acute effect of glucocorticoid deficiency (endogenous glucocorticoid has a small physiological inhibitory control over thyroid-stimulating hormone release) or associated autoimmune hypothyroidism. Thyroid function should be reassessed after glucocorticoid treatment has been established before considering thyroxine replacement.

Investigation

The diagnosis of adrenal insufficiency is established by demonstrating inappropriately low cortisol secretion, and is subsequently confirmed as primary or secondary by measurement of plasma ACTH. Other investigations are then directed at establishing the underlying cause. An undetectable serum cortisol is diagnostic. Morning serum cortisol concentrations (8–9 a.m.) of less than 100 nmol/L are strongly suggestive of adrenal insufficiency, whereas serum cortisol concentrations of greater than 600 nmol/L exclude the diagnosis in almost all cases. However, interpretation of cortisol values must always take into account the patient's condition, as relatively 'normal' levels for a healthy population may be inappropriate for individuals who are critically ill. Inappropriately low serum cortisol concentrations (especially during acute physical stress) in association with increased plasma ACTH concentrations determined simultaneously are usually diagnostic of primary adrenal insufficiency.

A short ACTH stimulation test is the key investigation and involves the intravenous (or intramuscular) administration of synthetic ACTH (synacthen 250 μg), with measurement of serum cortisol at baseline and 30 min after the injection. A rise in serum cortisol concentration after 30 min to a peak of 500–550 nmol/L or more (laboratories should be encouraged to establish their own reference range) is a normal response and excludes the diagnosis of primary adrenal insufficiency and almost all cases of secondary adrenal insufficiency. However, an important practice point is that falsely reassuring normal responses may occur in recent-onset secondary adrenal insufficiency in which the adrenal glands may not have atrophied and consequently retain their ACTH responsiveness. It is also worth noting that neither a 60-min measurement nor the 0- to 30-min increment in cortisol adds any value to the test. The test can be performed at any time of day, and there is no convincing evidence at present to support the use of a 'low' dose (1 μg) of synacthen in preference to 250 μg. It is important that steroid administration is not delayed to accommodate this test in sick patients; if dynamic testing is required, this can be performed at a later date when the patient's condition has stabilized.

After establishing the diagnosis of primary adrenal insufficiency, further investigations to determine the aetiology are indicated depending on clinical suspicion (see Box 5.1). Adrenal autoantibodies and computerized tomography (CT) imaging of the adrenals (Fig. 5.3) are usually recommended. In autoimmune adrenalitis, the glands are usually small and atrophic.

Treatment

Adrenal insufficiency is a potentially life-threatening condition, and treatment should be initiated as soon as the diagnosis is confirmed or as soon as suspected in a sick patient in hypotensive shock (Box 5.3).

Once the patient's condition has stabilized, the diagnosis has been confirmed and the patient is eating and drinking, parenteral glucocorticoid therapy can be tapered and converted to an oral maintenance dose. Patients with primary adrenal insufficiency require lifelong glucocorticoid and usually mineralocorticoid replacement therapy. Hydrocortisone is the treatment of choice, given in total daily doses of 15–30 mg. Doses are divided in twice-daily (e.g. 10 mg b.d.) or thrice-daily (e.g. 10 mg on waking, 5 mg at lunchtime and 5 mg around 6 p.m.) regimens. The longer-acting glucocorticoids prednisolone or dexamethasone can be used in equivalent doses (0.75 mg of dexamethasone = 5 mg of prednisolone = 20 mg of hydrocortisone), but there are often concerns regarding the risk of over-replacement, particularly with long-acting

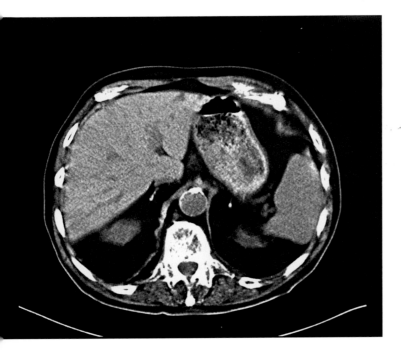

Figure 5.3
Computerized tomography (CT) imaging of adrenals in primary adrenal insufficiency. This CT scan shows evidence of small atrophic and calcified adrenal glands in an elderly man presenting with insidious adrenal failure. Atrophic calcified adrenal glands may occur following previous infections (e.g. tuberculosis), haemorrhage/ infarction or occasionally autoimmune destruction.

Box 5.3: Treatment of adrenal crisis

1. Draw blood samples for electrolytes, glucose, cortisol and adrenocorticotrophic hormone.
2. Fluids: large volumes of 0.9% saline are required to correct volume and sodium depletion.
3. Hydrocortisone: give bolus dose of 100 mg of hydrocortisone intravenously, followed by 100 mg intramuscularly or intravenously 6–8 hourly for the first 24–48 h. Double replacement doses (e.g. 20, 10 and 10 mg of hydrocortisone orally) can then be continued as the patient's condition stabilizes.
4. Mineralocorticoid: high-dose glucocorticoids provide sufficient mineralocorticoid effects during the initial stages of management. When glucocorticoids reach standard replacement doses, fludrocortisone 0.1 mg daily can be started (unnecessary in secondary adrenal failure).
5. Monitor and treat hypoglycaemia if present.
6. Suspect and treat precipitants (e.g. infection).

---

dexamethasone. Mineralocorticoid replacement therapy is required to minimize postural hypotension, prevent sodium loss and intravascular volume depletion, and correct hyperkalaemia. It is given in the form of fludrocortisone in a typical dose of 0.05–0.15 mg daily.

In women, the adrenal cortex is also the primary source of DHEA and DHEA sulphate. Some recent evidence suggests a role for DHEA replacement (given typically as 50 mg once daily) in women with primary adrenal insufficiency, with improvements noted in well-being and sexual function, but further research, especially in relation to long-term safety, is needed before this becomes standard therapy. Nevertheless, women who have significant symptoms of androgen deficiency can be offered a short-term trial of DHEA replacement.

There is ongoing controversy as to the most effective way of monitoring replacement therapy, achieving a balance of adequate glucocorticoid replacement on the one hand while avoiding over-replacement and the risk of long-term side-effects (e.g. weight gain, osteoporosis) on the other. Monitoring serum cortisol levels (e.g. hydrocortisone day curves) is unproven as an effective means of tailoring the hydrocortisone dose, and many clinicians are guided by simple clinical response and the patient's day-to-day symptoms. A history of frequent adrenal crisis may prompt a dose increment, while progressive weight gain may warrant a dose reduction. The maintenance dose of fludrocortisone should be titrated individually on the basis of postural blood pressure, serum electrolytes and measurement of plasma renin activity.

Intercurrent illness

During acute physical stress, cortisol requirements are higher. For minor illnesses or surgical procedures, the dose of glucocorticoid can be increased up to three times the usual maintenance dosage for a few days. During elective procedures (e.g. endoscopy), a single dose of 100 mg of hydrocortisone intravenously prior to the procedure should suffice. During major illness or surgery, high doses of glucocorticoid (e.g. 100 mg of intravenous or intramuscular hydrocortisone given 6–8 hourly) should be administered for a few days postoperatively or until resolution of illness.

Patient education

One of the important aspects of the management of chronic primary adrenal insufficiency is patient and family education. Patients should understand the reason for lifelong replacement therapy and the need to increase the dose of glucocorticoid during minor or major stress and to inject hydrocortisone in emergencies. It is prudent for centres to issue patients with emergency hydrocortisone injection packs, together with explanatory leaflets and advice on how to use them. Patients should also be encouraged to wear a MedicAlert bracelet or necklace and to carry a steroid card. Patient support groups such as the Pituitary Foundation (http://www.pituitary.org.uk) and the Addison's Disease Self Help Group (http://www.adshg.org.uk) may also prove useful resources.

CONGENITAL ADRENAL HYPERPLASIA IN ADULTS

Congenital adrenal hyperplasia (CAH) is a family of inherited disorders of adrenal steroidogenesis resulting from a deficiency of one of several enzymes necessary for normal steroid synthesis. The most common form of CAH, accounting for more than 90% of cases, is 21-hydroxylase deficiency, which is inherited in an autosomal recessive manner. 21-Hydroxylase deficiency occurs in two forms: classical and non-classical. Classical 21-hydroxylase deficiency is further divided into two types: salt wasting and simple virilizing. The second most common form of CAH is deficiency of the 11-β-hydroxylase enzyme, accounting for 5–8% of all cases.

The overall incidence of CAH in the general population depends on racial origin. In white populations, the carrier frequency of classical CAH is one in 60 and 3% for non-classical CAH, whereas in Ashkenazi Jews it is 19% for non-classical CAH.

In the common forms of CAH, the enzyme defect leads to a block in cortisol synthesis, impairing the cortisol-mediated feedback system. The resulting oversecretion of ACTH stimulates excessive synthesis of adrenal hormones in those pathways unimpaired by the enzyme deficiency and causes a build-up of precursors (e.g. 17-hydroxyprogesterone, 17-OHP, in 21-hydroxylase deficiency) in pathways blocked by the enzyme deficiency (see Fig. 5.1). The clinical symptoms of the three different forms of CAH result from the particular hormones that are deficient and those that are produced in excess. In 21-hydroxylase deficiency, the aldosterone and cortisol pathways are blocked and the androgen pathway, which does not involve 21-hydroxylation, is overstimulated, leading to virilization.

Clinical features

Classical 21-hydroxylase deficiency

The most prominent clinical feature of classical 21-hydroxylase deficiency (see also Ch. 2) is virilization of the female fetus, because it is exposed to excessive adrenal androgens secreted by the hyperplastic adrenal cortex from the third month of gestation onwards.

119

As a result, the external genitalia range from mildly ambiguous to completely virilized. Males with 21-hydroxylase deficiency do not exhibit genital abnormalities at birth. Lack of postnatal treatment in boys and girls results in continued exposure to excessive androgens, causing progressive penile or clitoral enlargement and the development of premature pubic and axillary hair. An early growth spurt is accompanied by premature epiphyseal fusion and ultimately short stature. Menstrual irregularity and secondary amenorrhoea commonly occur in inadequately treated adolescent girls. Some develop a clinical picture similar to polycystic ovarian syndrome, with hyperandrogenism, irregular menstrual bleeding, anovulation and polycystic ovaries. In male patients with classical CAH, the majority who have been adequately treated undergo normal pubertal development, have normal testicular function and have normal spermatogenesis and fertility. Salt wasting occurs in approximately three-quarters of classical 21-hydroxylase deficiency cases and results from aldosterone deficiency. Salt-wasting crises, which often occur in the neonatal period, are characterized by hyponatraemia, hyperkalaemia, metabolic acidosis and elevated plasma renin activity.

Non-classical 21-hydroxylase deficiency

Non-classical or late-onset 21-hydroxylase deficiency is caused by a partial deficiency of 21-hydroxylase and is more common than the classical form. It usually presents in girls around the onset of puberty or in early adult life with hirsutism, acne, oligomenorrhoea and subfertility. Genital ambiguity is not a feature. The clinical features overlap with those of polycystic ovarian syndrome, and non-classical CAH should be included in the differential diagnosis of this common condition. The diagnosis of non-classical CAH is based on the finding of elevated 17-OHP in association with hyperandrogenism (Box 5.4).

Management principles in CAH

In CAH, replacement therapy with corticosteroid (e.g. hydrocortisone, prednisolone, dexamethasone) in standard replacement doses is used to correct the deficiency in cortisol secretion, which will in turn suppress ACTH overproduction and consequent stimulation of the androgen pathway. This prevents further virilization, allowing normal growth and onset of puberty. A delicate balance must be struck between suppression of androgens and 17-OHP levels on the one hand and avoidance of glucocorticoid over-replacement on the other. Hydrocortisone is the corticosteroid of choice for children with CAH,

---

Box 5.4: Diagnosis of non-classical congenital adrenal hyperplasia

- Check basal 17-hydroxyprogesterone (17-OHP) (at 9 a.m. and during the follicular phase of the menstrual cycle):
  —if 17-OHP <5 nmol/L, diagnosis is excluded
  —if 17-OHP >15 nmol/L, diagnosis is very likely
  —if 17-OHP is 5–15 nmol/L, perform synacthen test with measurement of 17-OHP at 60 min.
- A postsynacthen 17-OHP level >45 nmol/L suggests non-classical congenital adrenal hyperplasia (most normal levels are <30 nmol/L).
- Mutational analysis of the 21-hydroxylase gene can confirm the diagnosis.

because of its short half-life and less propensity for over-replacement and suppression of normal growth. Salt wasters also require mineralocorticoid replacement therapy with fludrocortisone.

In paediatric practice, the principal therapeutic goal is centred on optimizing final height, whereas in adulthood the major aims are to:

- regulate hyperandrogenism
- restore fertility
- avoid glucocorticoid over-replacement.

Monitoring of treatment in adult CAH

The therapeutic strategy involves using the minimum effective glucocorticoid dose determined by clinical and biochemical parameters. Serum 17-OHP, testosterone, androstenedione and plasma renin activity are commonly used in the monitoring of adult CAH patients. Oversuppression of 17-OHP signals the risk of glucocorticoid overtreatment and suggests a need for dose reduction. In contrast, raised levels of 17-OHP, testosterone and androstenedione suggest glucocorticoid undertreatment. It has been suggested that an optimal glucocorticoid dose is that which fails to fully suppress 17-OHP but maintains androgens in the mid-normal range.

With regard to mineralocorticoid replacement, adults are generally less susceptible to salt wasting than children are, but fludrocortisone replacement is still required in salt wasters and requires monitoring. The tendency of some adults to develop rising blood pressure with age may lead to a need for dose reduction. Generally, plasma renin activity should be maintained in the upper normal range.

Although there are no data concerning fracture risk in CAH and no convincing evidence of reduced bone mineral density, there are justifiable concerns over bone health, given the need for long-term glucocorticoids. Unless there is raised clinical suspicion (e.g. clear history of chronic glucocorticoid excess), most authorities would not recommend routine measurements of bone density in young adults, but assessment of bone density in adults over 40 years of age is probably justified.

Although as yet there is no proven link between CAH and premature cardiovascular disease, there are several factors that might influence vascular risk in CAH, such as:

- increased adiposity
- hyperandrogenism in females
- glucocorticoid excess
- dyslipidaemia.

Further research in this area is required before specific recommendations can be made.

Fertility in CAH

With improved endocrine and reproductive care in specialized units, fertility and successful pregnancy is increasingly achievable in women with CAH. Reasons for reduced fertility in CAH include inadequate suppression of adrenal androgens, leading to ovulatory dysfunction often associated with polycystic ovaries; genital tract abnormalities, leading to unsatisfactory sexual intercourse; elevated progesterone levels in the follicular phase, leading to failure of implantation; and psychological problems commonly associated with the condition.

In a recent series from the Middlesex Hospital, UK, 11 out of 12 CAH women seeking fertility successfully conceived (spontaneously in five). Assisted reproductive techniques using gonadotrophins and clomiphene citrate have been used with success, and in a few very difficult cases bilateral adrenalectomy has led to successful conception and pregnancy outcome. Issues surrounding the management of CAH in pregnancy are discussed in Chapter 8.

Previously, the need for glucocorticoid treatment in adult men without salt-wasting disease was uncertain, and in some cases treatment was discontinued after attainment of final height, with patients being lost to long-term follow-up. However, there is now evidence that long-term control of CAH is important to preserve fertility. In addition, testicular abnormalities including adrenal rest tissue and impaired spermatogenesis have been reported in adult CAH men with inadequate adrenal suppression. It is therefore advisable that adult CAH men should have a testicular ultrasound after puberty and perhaps repeat ultrasound examinations on a 3- to 5-yearly basis. Evidence of adrenal rest tissue should prompt more effective adrenal androgen suppression with glucocorticoids, especially if fertility is desirable.

Management of non-classical CAH in adult women

In non-classical CAH in adulthood, there is a rationale to use low-dose glucocorticoids in order to suppress ACTH drive and improve oligomenorrhoea and symptoms of hyperandrogenism (e.g. hirsutism, acne). However, conventional antiandrogens with oral oestrogens can be used as an alternative, as in the management of hyperandrogenism associated with polycystic ovarian syndrome.

ADRENAL CUSHING'S SYNDROME

Cushing's syndrome results from chronic exposure to excessive levels of glucocorticoids (hypercortisolism). Although the condition is relatively rare, the overlap of many of its physical manifestations (obesity, hypertension, diabetes) with clinical states such as polycystic ovary syndrome and type 2 diabetes means that screening for Cushing's syndrome is becoming increasingly common. In addition, increased awareness has meant that the diagnosis is often considered before the development of the more classical signs and symptoms. When severe and untreated, hypercortisolism is associated with a high mortality, approaching 50% at 5 years. However, more subtle cortisol excess may also lead to significant morbidity, having important effects on glucose metabolism, blood pressure and cardiovascular risk. A description of subclinical Cushing's syndrome in relation to adrenal incidentalomas is given later in this chapter.

Hypercortisolism is either ACTH-dependent or ACTH-independent (Table 5.1). Adrenal-driven disease is due to excessive autonomous cortisol secretion from an adrenal adenoma or carcinoma. Of the ACTH-dependent forms, pituitary-dependent hypercortisolism (Cushing's disease) accounts for the majority of cases, with ectopic ACTH production from a variety of tumour types forming the remainder. The investigation and management of Cushing's disease is described in Chapter 1.

The clinical features and investigation of hypercortisolism are described fully in Chapter 1. In ACTH-independent Cushing's syndrome, features of hyperandrogenism with or without virilization may be prominent due to excessive adrenal androgen production by an adrenal adenoma or carcinoma. Severe hirsutism and virilization, particularly when associated with a large adrenal tumour (often >10 cm), strongly suggest an adrenal carcinoma.

Treatment

For adrenal adenomas, unilateral adrenalectomy (open or, more commonly nowadays, laparoscopic) is the definitive treatment and is curative in most cases, with recurrence unlikely. Temporary adrenal insufficiency usually occurs postoperatively due to prior inhibition of ACTH by the high circulating glucocorticoid concentrations, with consequent suppression of the unaffected contralateral adrenal gland. Glucocorticoid replacement is therefore needed and may be required for several months or years (in a small proportion, recovery does not ensue and patients require lifelong replacement). This can be given as either hydrocortisone or prednisolone, although the latter has the advantage of allowing greater fine tuning of dose reduction (it is available in 1-mg doses, whereas the smallest dose of hydrocortisone tablet is 10 mg) as the gland recovers function. Recovery of function should be confirmed by periodic synacthen tests a month after any glucocorticoid dose reduction. For ACTH-independent bilateral adrenal hyperplasia, bilateral adrenalectomy is often indicated, necessitating lifelong glucocorticoid and mineralocorticoid replacement.

Table 5.1: Causes and frequency of endogenous Cushing's syndrome

	Frequency (%)
ACTH-dependent	
Pituitary-dependent Cushing's syndrome (Cushing's disease)	68
Ectopic ACTH syndrome	12
Ectopic corticotrophin-releasing hormone syndrome	<1
ACTH-independent	
Adrenal adenoma	10
Adrenal carcinoma	8
Macronodular adrenal hyperplasia	1
Pigmented micronodular adrenal hyperplasia	1

ACTH, adrenocorticotrophic hormone.

Adrenal cancer carries a poor prognosis, with disease-free survival of around 30% at 5 years. Open surgery aimed at complete resection is the treatment of choice, but local recurrence is common. Surgery also plays a role in combating local tumour recurrence and metastases. Patients for whom surgery is unsuccessful or not possible receive medical therapy, usually with a combination of adrenolytic and cytotoxic agents. Mitotane remains the drug of choice, but other agents including etoposide, doxorubicin and cisplatin are under evaluation in clinical trials. Adrenolytic agents including metyrapone, ketoconazole and aminoglutethimide are indicated for uncontrolled hypercortisolism.

PRIMARY ALDOSTERONISM AND MINERALOCORTICOID EXCESS

Primary aldosteronism (PA) due to either an aldosterone-producing adenoma (Conn's syndrome) or adrenal hyperplasia (usually bilateral) is the commonest form of endocrine hypertension in which aldosterone production is inappropriate and at least partially independent of the renin–angiotensin system. PA was previously believed to account for less than 1% of hypertensive patients, and hypokalaemia was considered a prerequisite for pursuing the diagnosis. However, while classical Conn's syndrome with hypertension, hypokalaemic alkalosis and an adrenal adenoma is relatively rare, recent studies utilizing the plasma aldosterone : renin ratio (ARR) (suppressed renin and elevated aldosterone suggestive of PA) in unselected hypertensive populations have reported a much higher prevalence of the condition of between 5 and 13%, with hyperplasia rather than adenoma accounting for the majority. Despite this, most authorities would not recommend screening with ARR in all hypertensive patients, but targeted screening should be adopted (see Fig. 5.4). A random ARR of >25–30 (assuming aldosterone is expressed as ng/dl and renin as ng/ml/h) is now considered a sensitive screening test for the diagnosis of PA. In the event of a positive screening test, confirmatory tests are generally recommended to establish the diagnosis of PA before proceeding to imaging.

Suggested algorithms for the investigation of endocrine hypertension and PA are shown in Figures 5.4 and 5.5. Although a number of antihypertensive drugs can affect the ARR (especially beta blockers, which suppress plasma renin activity; Table 5.2), it is usually justifiable to screen patients while on treatment, with the exception of aldosterone receptor antagonists (e.g. spironolactone, eplerenone). Hypokalaemia should also be corrected, as it directly inhibits aldosterone release. In the event of a positive ratio, antihypertensive therapy is usually modified during confirmatory tests (notably beta blockers are discontinued; ACE inhibitors often give a false negative ARR, as they suppress aldosterone, so a positive ratio on ACE inhibitors may be particularly suggestive of PA and they probably do not need to be discontinued in practice). A number of dynamic tests have been used to confirm the diagnosis, with the purpose of demonstrating autonomy and non-suppressibility of aldosterone production. Examples are the fludrocortisone suppression test, postcaptopril test and salt-loading tests (intravenous or oral). In the intravenous saline suppression test, upright plasma aldosterone is measured before and again supine after administering 500 mL of 0.9%

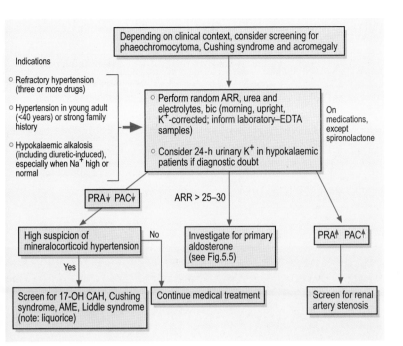

Figure 5.4
The investigation of endocrine hypertension. AME, apparent mineralocorticoid excess; ARR, aldosterone : renin ratio; CAH, congenital adrenal hyperplasia; PAC, plasma aldosterone concentration; PRA, plasma renin activity.

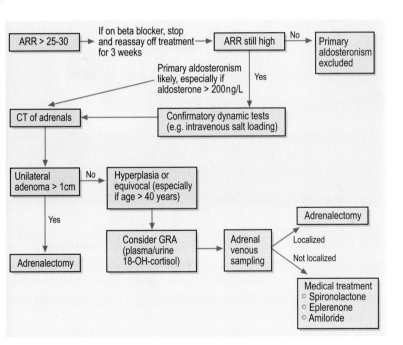

Figure 5.5
The investigation of primary aldosteronism. ARR, aldosterone : renin ratio; CT, computerized tomography; GRA, glucocorticoid-remediable aldosteronism.

saline over 4 h. PA is confirmed if aldosterone levels fail to suppress below 60 ng/L. Salt-loading and fludrocortisone tests are contraindicated in heart failure. Thin-slice adrenal CT is the investigation of choice to determine the presence of small adrenal adenomas or hyperplasia (Fig. 5.6). If an adrenal tumour is identified in a patient with biochemically proven PA and the contralateral adrenal gland is anatomically normal, no further

Table 5.2: Effects of antihypertensive medications on the aldosterone:renin ratio

Drug	Effect on renin	Effect on aldosterone
Spironolactone[a]	Increase	Increase
Beta blockers	Decrease	Decrease
Angiotensin-converting enzyme inhibitors	Increase	Decrease
Angiotensin receptor blockers	Increase	Decrease
Diuretics	Increase	Decrease
Alpha blockers	No effect	No effect
Calcium channel blockers	Usually no effect	Usually no effect

[a]A 4- to 6-week washout period is required to reverse effects (approximately 2 weeks for other drugs).

Figure 5.6
Bilateral adrenal hyperplasia. Abdominal computerized tomography scan showing evidence of diffuse bilateral adrenal enlargement (particularly on the left – see arrow) suggestive of hyperplasia in a patient with primary aldosteronism.

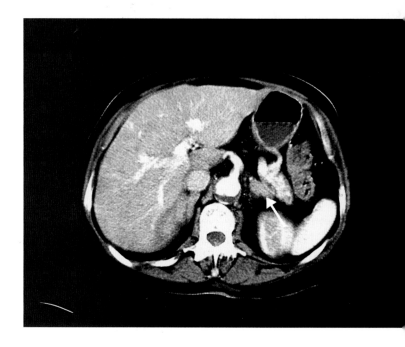

evaluation is usually needed and surgery is recommended (especially in individuals below the age of 40 with lesions >1 cm). In equivocal cases when surgical cure is considered a possibility, adrenal vein sampling is the investigation of choice and, although technically difficult (cannulation of the right adrenal vein is often challenging), is considered the gold standard in differentiating unilateral from bilateral aldosterone excess.

Treatment

Laparoscopic adrenalectomy is the treatment of choice in PA due to an adrenal adenoma, with hypertension cure rates of approximately 70%. Cure is less likely in older individuals and those with a family history of hypertension. Bilateral adrenal hyperplasia is treated medically with the use of aldosterone receptor antagonists, usually spironolactone (50–400 mg daily) or more recently eplerenone. While effective for controlling blood pressure and hypokalaemia, the use of spironolactone is limited by side-effects (usually at doses >100 mg/day), especially in male patients, who may develop gynaecomastia. Eplerenone is an alternative in such patients, as is the potassium-sparing diuretic amiloride.

Other mineralocorticoid excess states

Rarely, the clinical syndrome of mineralocorticoid hypertension is caused by mechanisms other than hyperaldosteronism. These should be considered in the presence of hypokalaemic hypertension associated with suppressed renin and aldosterone levels that are normal or reduced.

Glucocorticoid-remediable aldosteronism

Glucocorticoid-remediable aldosteronism (GRA) is an autosomal dominant disorder characterized by a chimeric duplication in which a portion of the 11-β-hydroxylase gene (regulated by ACTH) is fused to the coding sequence of the aldosterone synthase gene. In this setting, aldosterone synthesis comes under ACTH control. This condition should be considered in younger individuals with early-onset hypertension in the setting of a suppressed plasma renin activity. A strong family history of early cerebral haemorrhage (<35 years) should also raise suspicion for GRA. The diagnosis is supported by the finding of marked elevations of the adrenal-derived hybrid steroid 18-hydroxy cortisol in plasma and urine. Genetic testing to identify the presence of the gene duplication in GRA is also now possible to confirm the diagnosis.

Glucocorticoid-remediable aldosteronism can be successfully treated by turning off the ACTH drive with low doses of glucocorticoids such as dexamethasone. Spironolactone, eplerenone and amiloride are also effective treatments for hypertension in GRA and are alternatives to glucocorticoid suppression.

The syndrome of apparent mineralocorticoid excess

The syndrome of apparent mineralocorticoid excess results from abnormal activation of the mineralocorticoid receptor in the kidney by cortisol. The mineralocorticoid receptor is usually protected from excessive activation by cortisol (which circulates in concentrations several orders of magnitude greater than aldosterone) by a key regulatory enzyme in the kidney, 11-β-hydroxysteroid dehydrogenase type 2 (11βHSD2). Deficiency of 11βHSD2 from inactivating mutations or inhibition by excessive liquorice or grapefruit consumption leads to apparent mineralocorticoid excess.

A similar scenario may occur in severe Cushing's syndrome (e.g. from ectopic ACTH production) when very high circulating concentrations of cortisol saturate the 11βHSD2 enzyme system and expose the mineralocorticoid receptor to active cortisol, resulting in hypertension and hypokalaemia.

The diagnosis is supported by the finding of an elevated urinary free tetrahydrocortisol:tetrahydrocortisone ratio in a timed collection. Genetic testing is required in suspected inherited cases. Treatment consists of spironolactone, amiloride or eplerenone.

Liddle's syndrome

Liddle's syndrome is a rare autosomal dominant condition caused by an activating mutation of the renal epithelial sodium channel, resulting in its constitutive activation and hence excessive sodium reabsorption and hypokalaemic hypertension. The diagnosis is suggested by the exclusion of other causes of mineralocorticoid hypertension and identification of a mutation affecting the epithelial sodium channel. Treatment is with amiloride, which acts on the sodium channel directly.

RENAL TUBULAR DISORDERS

In the investigation of the hypokalaemic patient, disorders of tubular function should be considered in the differential diagnosis. In Bartter syndrome and Gitelman syndrome, there is evidence of hypokalaemic alkalosis and activation of the renin–angiotensin system, but importantly in the absence of hypertension. Gitelman syndrome, which represents a less severe phenotype than Bartter syndrome, may present in adulthood and is caused by a genetic abnormality leading to loss of function in the thiazide-sensitive sodium chloride transporter of the distal tubule. This leads to salt wasting, hypovolaemia and hypokalaemia, often with hypomagnesaemia and hypocalciuria. Investigation is by measurement of appropriate urinary electrolyte excretion, and treatment is with potassium and magnesium supplementation.

PHAEOCHROMOCYTOMA

Phaeochromocytomas are catecholamine-secreting tumours occurring in approximately 0.1% of patients with sustained hypertension. In about 90% of cases, they arise from the adrenal medulla, and in the remaining 10% from extra-adrenal chromaffin tissue (paragangliomas). Although most phaeochromocytomas are sporadic, increasingly a familial basis for these tumours is recognized, with germline mutations in VHL, RET or the recently recognized succinate dehydrogenase gene family (SDHB and SDHD), accounting for up to 25% of apparently sporadic disease (Table 5.3). Sporadic phaeochromocytomas are usually unilateral, while familial phaeochromocytomas are often bilateral and may be extra-adrenal. Approximately 10–20% of tumours are malignant, characterized by local invasion or distant metastases. The secretory products from phaeochromocytomas are principally noradrenaline (norepinephrine) and adrenaline (epinephrine) (and their metabolites) and occasionally dopamine. Rarely, other co-produced peptide hormones including ACTH, vasoactive intestinal peptide, growth hormone-releasing hormone and parathyroid hormone produce clinical manifestations of the relevant hormone excess.

Table 5.3: Familial syndromes and phaeochromocytoma

Syndrome	Features
von Hippel–Lindau syndrome	Renal cell carcinoma, cerebellar haemangioblastoma, retinal and spinal angiomas
Multiple endocrine neoplasia types 2a and 2b	Hyperparathyroidism, medullary thyroid carcinoma (marfanoid habitus and mucosal neuromas in multiple endocrine neoplasia type 2b)
Neurofibromatosis type 1	Phaeochromocytoma prevalence in this disorder is about 1%
Succinate dehydrogenase subunit D (SDHD) and subunit B (SDHB) mutations	Familial paragangliomas in head, neck and abdomen

Clinical features and investigation

Phaeochromocytomas are characterized by clinical signs and symptoms that result from the metabolic and haemodynamic actions of circulating catecholamines, including noradrenaline, adrenaline and dopamine. The more common presenting symptoms include:

- sustained or paroxysmal hypertension (>90%)
- headache (90%)
- sweating (60–70%)
- pallor (30%)
- palpitations (30%).

A variety of other symptoms may occur, including anxiety, nervousness, panic attacks, pyrexia and postural hypotension due to plasma volume contraction. The clinical presentation in individual cases depends on the predominant catecholamine released from the tumour, together with its pattern of release. Noradrenaline-secreting tumours tend to cause sustained hypertension, whereas tumours secreting significant amounts of adrenaline and noradrenaline often cause episodic hypertension. Pure adrenaline- and dopamine-secreting tumours can cause hypotension.

An untreated phaeochromocytoma is a potentially lethal condition associated with a variety of complications, including:

- hypertensive crisis
- encephalopathy
- ventricular arrhythmias
- left ventricular failure
- pulmonary oedema and hyperglycaemia.

Notable precipitators of hypertensive crises in patients with phaeochromocytoma include radiographic contrast media, dopamine antagonists, opiates, tricyclic antidepressants and cocaine.

patients must be protected from catecholamine excess by pharmacological alpha and beta blockade. Alpha blockade must be commenced prior to beta blockade to avoid unopposed α-adrenergic stimulation and a risk of a hypertensive crisis. Conventionally, the alpha blocker phenoxybenzamine (starting dose 10 mg b.d., increased to 20 mg q.d.s. or more until blood pressure is adequately controlled or side-effects, e.g. nasal stuffiness or postural hypotension, become dose-limiting) is used, followed by a non-selective beta blocker such as propranolol to oppose catecholamine-induced arrhythmias and reflex tachycardias often associated with alpha blockade. Patients with a contraindication to beta blockade may be treated with a rate-limiting calcium channel antagonist; some centres are now using these as sole agents in pre- and perioperative preparation.

Careful anaesthetic assessment by an experienced anaesthetist is required prior to surgery, because of the risk of major fluctuations in blood pressure and the risk of cardiac arrhythmias. Perioperative hypertensive crises may be treated with intravenous phentolamine or sodium nitroprusside, and arrhythmias controlled with intravenous esmolol or propranolol. Intra- or postoperative hypotension following resection of the tumour usually responds to fluid replacement.

Surgical removal of intra-adrenal phaeochromocytomas is usually successfully carried out either laparoscopically or, for larger or bilateral tumours, by open surgery. Hypertension is cured in the majority of patients. Long-term follow-up is advised, and cure is assessed by monitoring 24-h urinary catecholamines. Five-year survival for apparently benign tumours is 96%, and the recurrence rate is less than 10%. Malignant phaeochromocytoma may be treated with systemic chemotherapy and/or iodine-131 MIBG therapy. In patients with metastatic phaeochromocytoma, average life expectancy is about 5 years from the time of initial diagnosis.

ADRENAL INCIDENTALOMAS

Modern imaging techniques, particularly CT and MRI, enable the detection of adrenal tumours with high sensitivity. Given that autopsy studies reveal a relatively high incidence of adrenal nodules (approximately 3–7% over the age of 50), it is not surprising that, with the widespread and increasing use of these imaging techniques in many areas of medicine, the detection of incidentally discovered adrenal masses is becoming a common clinical problem. An incidentally detected adrenal mass or incidentaloma is defined as an adrenal tumour not suspected prior to the imaging procedure that led to its discovery. Therefore, by definition, clinical symptoms and/or signs of an adrenal tumour must not precede the diagnosis of an incidentally detected adrenal mass. The clinical problems that should be addressed after the finding of an incidentaloma are as follows:

- Is it an adrenal or extra-adrenal mass?
- Is the adrenal mass a metastasis of an unknown or a known primary tumour?
- Is the adrenal mass hormonally active?
- Is there evidence of adrenocortical carcinoma?

At the time of diagnosis, up to 20% of all incidentalomas may be endocrinologically active. The likelihood that an incidentaloma is active increases with increasing size of the lesion, with the exception of aldosterone-producing adenomas associated with hypertension, which are often small (<1 cm). Larger tumours are also more likely to be malignant, with the risk being high for lesions >6 cm in diameter.

Management of adrenal incidentalomas

A suggested algorithm for the investigation and management of incidentalomas is shown in Figure 5.8. Adrenalectomy is indicated if the lesion is hormonally active, although controversy exists in milder cases of subclinical Cushing's syndrome (see below). Surgery is definitely indicated for lesions >6 cm. Hormonally inactive lesions that are <4 cm are normally managed conservatively, but there remains some uncertainty for lesions of 4–6 cm, with the option of either surgery or conservative management and surveillance if radiological features are in favour of a benign lesion. In all cases in which surgery is not undertaken, repeat imaging should be performed at 6–12 months following initial imaging. During follow-up, all tumours demonstrating significant growth, showing radiological features favouring malignancy or exhibiting evidence of hormonal activity should be removed. If the lesion is unchanged in size, long-term follow-up is considered unnecessary by some authorities, but long-term prospective studies are currently lacking.

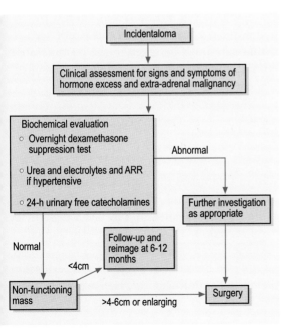

Figure 5.8
Suggested work-up for adrenal incidentalomas. ARR, aldosterone:renin ratio.

> **Box 5.7: Criteria for the diagnosis of subclinical Cushing's syndrome**
>
> - No clinical signs of hormone excess (i.e. truncal obesity, thin extremities with myopathy, moon face and cutaneous purple striae) should be present, *and*
> - at least two abnormalities in hypothalamic–pituitary–adrenal axis function:
>   —failure to suppress cortisol with dexamethasone (standard 48-h low-dose test) (mandatory)
>   —loss of normal circadian rhythm
>   —elevated urinary free cortisol
>   —low morning adrenocorticotrophic hormone

SUBCLINICAL CUSHING'S SYNDROME

Some patients with incidentally discovered adrenal adenomas display varying degrees of autonomous cortisol secretion with altered pituitary ACTH negative feedback sensitivity, a condition that has been defined as subclinical Cushing's syndrome. It is increasingly recognized with adrenal incidentalomas and is characterized by mild, autonomous hypercortisolaemia without specific clinical signs of cortisol excess. An increased prevalence of hypertension, obesity and impaired glucose tolerance has been described in subclinical Cushing's syndrome, suggesting parallels with the metabolic syndrome. No universally accepted definition of this diagnosis exists, but suggested criteria are given in Box 5.7. The natural history of subclinical Cushing's syndrome remains unclear, but most would now advocate adrenalectomy in clear-cut cases associated with an identifiable adrenal lesion. Some centres find cholesterol scintigraphy (iodocholesterol or selenocholesterol scan) performed under dexamethasone suppression a useful test to confirm autonomous hyperfunction of a small adrenal mass, although this is not routinely performed. It must be emphasized that care must be taken in the postoperative period, as temporary suppression of the contralateral adrenal may precipitate adrenal insufficiency necessitating corticosteroid replacement.

GLUCOCORTICOID RESISTANCE

Glucocorticoid resistance is a very rare condition that arises due to mutations (inherited or sporadic) in the glucocorticoid receptor-α gene. Because of impaired hypothalamic–pituitary sensitivity to cortisol, the hypothalamic–pituitary–adrenal axis has a higher 'set point', leading to increased ACTH and cortisol secretion, although diurnal rhythmicity is preserved. Patients are not cushingoid due to generalized tissue resistance to glucocorticoids, but mineralocorticoid excess may be present, giving rise to hypertension and hypokalaemia. Female patients may develop hyperandrogenism, menstrual irregularity, subfertility and polycystic ovaries. Treatment with a low dose of dexamethasone may be effective.

Further reading

Arlt W, Callies F, van Vlijmen JC et al. 1999 Dehydroepiandrosterone replacement in women with adrenal insufficiency. New Engl J Med 341: 1013–1020

Arnaldi G, Angeli A, Atkinson AB 2003 Diagnosis and complications of Cushing's syndrome: a consensus statement. J Clin Endocrinol Metab 88: 5593–5602

Bravo EL, Tagle R 2003 Pheochromocytoma: state of the art and future prospects. Endocr Rev 24: 539–553

Dluhy RG, Lifton RP 1999 Glucocorticoid-remediable aldosteronism. J Clin Endocrinol Metab 84: 4341–4344

Grinspoon SK, Biller BM 1994 Laboratory assessment of adrenal insufficiency. J Clin Endocrinol Metab 79: 923–931

Kloos RT, Gross MD, Francis IR et al. 1995 Incidentally discovered adrenal masses. Endocr Rev 16: 460–484

Lenders JW et al. 2002 Biochemical diagnosis of pheochromocytoma: which test is best? JAMA 287: 1427–1434

Nadar S, Lip GYH, Beevers G 2003 Primary aldosteronism. Ann Clin Biochem 40: 439–452

Newell-Price J, Trainer P, Besser M et al. 1998 The diagnosis and differential diagnosis of Cushing's syndrome and pseudo-Cushing's states. Endocr Rev 19: 647–672

Oelkers W 1996 Current concepts: adrenal insufficiency. New Engl J Med 335: 1206–1212

Rossi R, Tauchmanova L, Luciano A et al. 2000 Subclinical Cushing's syndrome in patients with adrenal incidentaloma: clinical and biochemical features. J Clin Endocrinol Metab 85: 1440–1448

White PC, Speiser PW 2000 Congenital adrenal hyperplasia due to 21-hydroxylase deficiency. Endocr Rev 21: 245–291

Young WF 2003 Minireview: primary aldosteronism – changing concepts in diagnosis and treatment. J Clin Endocrinol Metab 144: 2208–2213

SELF-ASSESSMENT

Patient 1

A 22-year-old man presents to the accident and emergency department after collapsing with abdominal pains, vomiting and diarrhoea. He has been unwell for several days with anorexia, weight loss and fever, having recently returned from a holiday abroad in the Mediterranean. Examination findings reveal evidence of hypovolaemic shock, with tachycardia, hypotension and cool peripheries. There is diffuse abdominal tenderness. Initial investigations reveal serum sodium of 126 mmol/L, potassium of 4.8 mmol/L and urea of 14 mmol/L. White blood count shows a neutrophilia, and C-reactive protein is elevated. The admitting doctor suspects adrenal failure.

Questions
1. What investigations are required to confirm or exclude the diagnosis of adrenal failure, and what other immediate investigations should be undertaken?
2. Describe the initial steps required in the treatment of this patient.
3. What subsequent investigations should be considered to establish the aetiology of adrenal insufficiency in this case?

Answers
1. There are a number of differential diagnoses in this case. However, the presenting features of predominantly gastrointestinal and abdominal symptoms (often mimicking an acute abdomen), together with hypovolaemic shock, hyponatraemia and raised urea, are characteristic of an adrenal crisis. Other urgent investigations required include blood glucose, blood and urine cultures to look for precipitating infection, and radiographs of chest and abdomen to investigate other potential causes or precipitants. Evidence of skin hyperpigmentation would be suggestive of primary adrenal failure, although this may be difficult to distinguish from tanned skin due to sun exposure. Blood samples should be immediately drawn for cortisol and ACTH prior to administration of steroids. Liaison with the biochemistry laboratory is required to ensure adequate collection and processing of plasma ACTH. Following collection of the above samples, potentially life-saving administration of steroids should not be delayed while results are awaited. In the above case, serum cortisol was 45 nmol/L and diagnostic of adrenal failure in the clinical setting. Subsequently, a raised plasma ACTH of 380 ng/L (0–40 ng/L) confirmed the diagnosis of primary adrenal failure.
2. Adrenal crisis is a life-threatening medical emergency and should be managed in a critical care setting with adequate resuscitation and monitoring facilities. After collection of initial blood samples, high-dose parenteral steroids (e.g. hydrocortisone 100 mg intravenous bolus followed by 100 mg 6–8 hourly intravenously or intramuscularly) should be administered for the first 24–48 h. Specific mineralocorticoid replacement is not required initially, as high-dose glucocorticoids will exert sufficient mineralocorticoid effects. Large volumes of intravenous 0.9% saline are required, and 10% dextrose in addition if hypoglycaemia is present. If there

is suspicion of underlying infection, as in this case, broad-spectrum intravenous antibiotics should be administered after appropriate cultures are taken.

3. After establishing the diagnosis of primary adrenal failure, CT imaging of the adrenals should be undertaken. In the UK, autoimmune adrenalitis is the commonest cause and is usually associated with atrophic adrenal gland appearances. Adrenal autoantibodies, if identified, confirm the diagnosis. In adolescent or young adult male patients, very long chain fatty acids should also be checked to screen for the rare condition of adrenoleucodystrophy. Screening for other associated immune-mediated conditions, including hypothyroidism, hypoparathyroidism, hypogonadism, pernicious anaemia and type 1 diabetes, should also be undertaken.

Patient 2

A 42-year-old woman is referred with refractory hypertension. Hypertension had been diagnosed 2 years earlier, with blood pressure recordings of around 170/100 mmHg. At the time, urea and electrolytes were within normal limits and urine dipstick was negative. She had been commenced on lisinopril, but blood pressure remained elevated. Shortly before referral, her general practitioner had commenced a thiazide diuretic. Repeat blood tests revealed potassium of 2.9 mmol/L, sodium of 143 mmol/L and normal urea and creatinine. The patient was seen by another physician colleague who, suspecting an adrenal disorder, requested a CT scan of the adrenals. The scan demonstrates the presence of a 1.8-cm lesion within the left adrenal gland but also a suspicion of a smaller 0.8-cm lesion within the right adrenal gland. She is referred to the endocrine service.

Questions
1. What diagnostic steps are required to confirm a diagnosis of PA?
2. What further investigation should be considered to assess whether adrenal surgery is indicated?
3. What therapeutic measures should be undertaken prior to surgery?

Answers
1. Secondary causes of hypertension – including the most common form of endocrine hypertension, PA – should always be considered in relatively young patients with refractory hypertension, including those who are normokalaemic. The fall in serum potassium after commencing a thiazide diuretic, together with serum sodium in the upper half of the normal range, increases the clinical suspicion. However, in this case biochemical confirmation of PA should have been made prior to imaging. An ARR is the screening investigation of choice and can be performed while on the above medications, both of which tend to lower the ratio (although it would be prudent in this case to withdraw the diuretic because of hypokalaemia). In the event of a negative test and if clinical suspicion remains, repeat testing can be arranged after discontinuing current medication and substituting with an alpha blocker if blood pressure rises. If the ARR is raised, a confirmatory test such as salt loading should be considered prior to adrenal imaging.

137

2. In the present case, the finding of bilateral lesions complicates the decision with regards to the possibility of surgery. Adrenalectomy is indicated only if aldosterone excess is shown to be unilateral; if bilateral secretion is demonstrated, long-term medical therapy with aldosterone blockade is the treatment of choice. The investigation of choice and most reliable method of determining the source of aldosterone excess is adrenal venous sampling. In the present case, adrenal venous sampling was successfully undertaken and demonstrated significant aldosterone excess on the left side relative to the right (aldosterone:cortisol ratio on the left more than four times the ratio from the right).

3. Laparoscopic left adrenalectomy was arranged. It is desirable to achieve adequate blood pressure control and correction of hypokalaemia prior to surgery. This is usually achieved with the preoperative use of an aldosterone blocker (e.g. spironolactone), with additional potassium supplements and other antihypertensive medication as required. Aldosterone blockers should be discontinued postoperatively to avoid possible mineralocorticoid deficiency.

Endocrine gonadal disease

J. Platts

ANATOMY AND PHYSIOLOGY

The ovary

The ovary consists of four cell types: germ cells, granulosa cells, theca cells and support cells. In embryonic life, germ cells migrate to the urogenital ridge, where they multiply at 5 weeks' gestation to form the primitive gonad. Oogonia are surrounded by granulosa cells to form a primordial follicle, and 3.5 million of these exist by 20 weeks' gestation. Two-thirds are destroyed in the last trimester, so that 1 million ova are present in each ovary at birth. This number declines to 300000 at puberty and 10000 at age 40, with a dramatic decline thereafter. Only 500 are utilized in ovulation.

The granulosa cells surrounding the primary follicle multiply to form the secondary follicle, and the outer layer become theca cells and develop luteinizing hormone (LH) receptors. Secondary follicles undergo changes to become tertiary or graafian follicles, which will release the oocyte into the fallopian tube and be transformed into the corpus luteum.

Ovulation comprises a complex sequence of events involving LH, follicle-stimulating hormone (FSH) and feedback mechanisms (Fig. 6.1).

Follicle-stimulating hormone rises at the end of the cycle in response to falling sex hormone levels. The rise in FSH stimulates development of early tertiary follicles. Androgens are produced from the theca cells in response to LH. The granulosa cells produce oestrogens from androgens as a result of aromatase activity. The oestrogen levels peak at days 10–12 and lead to a fall in FSH. The rising oestradiol causes a surge of LH; this triggers ovulation, and the remaining follicle forms the corpus luteum. The LH surge causes the theca cells to produce progesterone instead of androgen, and the granulosa cells also produce progesterone at this time. Inhibin inhibits FSH and enhances the effect of the sex steroids.

The hypothalamic–pituitary unit must be able to generate a pulsatile secretion of gonadotrophin-releasing hormone (GnRH) at a minimum frequency of one per hour to allow FSH to exceed the threshold to alter the granulosa cells to allow them to respond

Figure 6.1
Hormonal fluctuations of the menstrual cycle. FSH,
follicle-stimulating hormone; LH, luteinizing hormone.

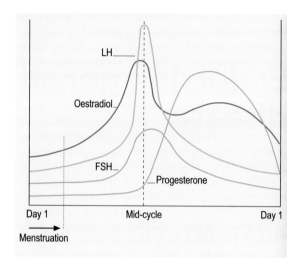

to LH. The ovary can produce oestrogen at a lower GnRH pulse frequency but ovulation will not occur, as the pituitary must be primed at a pulse rate of one per hour for a few days to respond to oestrogen with an ovulatory surge of LH.

If no fertilization occurs, the corpus luteum degenerates, oestrogen and progesterone levels fall and menstruation occurs. If fertilization occurs, progesterone levels are maintained by the corpus luteum, under the influence of human chorionic gonadotrophin (hCG), until the placenta takes over this function and the endometrial lining is maintained to allow implantation of the blastocyst.

The testis

The testis has two predominant groups of functional cells: the Leydig cells and the seminiferous tubules. Leydig cells produce testosterone under the influence of LH, and the seminiferous tubules are responsible for spermatogenesis. Each testis contains 600–900 seminiferous tubules occupying 85–90% of the volume of the testis. Sertoli cells extend from the basement membrane of the seminiferous tubules deep into the lumen; they are nursing cells for spermatids and spermatozoa until they are released into the epididymis. Sertoli cells secrete fluid and electrolytes under the control of FSH and testosterone.

At 6 weeks' gestation, the bipotential gonad is programmed to become a testis. The differentiated testis secretes antimüllerian hormone, which induces atrophy of the müllerian duct (which would otherwise form the uterus and fallopian tubes in the absence of antimüllerian hormone, regardless of genetic gender). Leydig cells appear at day 60. Testosterone organizes the wolffian duct into epididymis, vas deferens, seminal vesicle and adrenal gland structures, and by 16 weeks the fetus has adult male testosterone levels. Dihydrotestosterone develops male external genitalia, causing growth of the genital protruberance, fusion of the genital folds and labia, and differentiation of the prostate (see Ch. 2).

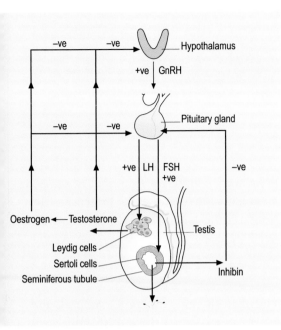

Figure 6.2
Regulation of testicular function. +ve, positive stimulation; -ve, negative feedback; FSH, follicle-stimulating hormone; GnRH, gonadotrophin-releasing hormone; LH, luteinizing hormone.

Spermatogenesis is under the control of FSH. As spermatogonia migrate and develop to become spermatids then spermatozoa, the Sertoli cells provide nutrients and growth factors. This takes 72 days. The Sertoli cells are essential for spermatogenesis, but the exact functions and mechanisms of interaction between Sertoli cells and spermatids and spermatozoa are unknown; there is a blood–testis barrier, and the composition of the fluid in the tubules is different from other body fluids (such as interstitial fluid) and controlled by the Sertoli cells. The spermatozoa then pass through the epididymis, vas deferens and ejaculatory ducts. Sertoli cells secrete inhibin, which inhibits FSH production. The relationship between these cells and hormones is summarized in Figure 6.2.

The parent substance of testosterone biosynthesis is cholesterol, which is converted to pregnenolone and, via less biologically active dehydroepiandrosterone and androstenediol, to androstenedione and testosterone. Testosterone is largely protein-bound (60% to sex hormone-binding globulin, SHBG, and 38% to albumin), with 2% circulating as biologically active free testosterone. Testosterone is metabolized to dihydrotestosterone and 17-β-oestradiol. Oestradiol is produced by extratesticular aromatization of testosterone and androstenedione.

ASSESSMENT OF GONADAL FUNCTION

This must be performed in the context of the presenting complaint: the assessment of a woman with oligomenorrhoea and normal oestrogen will be different from that of someone with oligomenorrhoea and low oestrogen. Similarly, assessment of primary

Table 6.1: The gonadotrophin-releasing hormone test

Time from administration of gonadotrophin-releasing hormone (min)	Luteinizing hormone (mU/L)	Follicle-stimulating hormone (mU/L)
20	13–58	1–7
60	11–48	1–5

gonadal failure (raised gonadotrophins) will be entirely different from that of someone with secondary gonadal failure (low or normal gonadotrophins in the presence of low testosterone or oestradiol). Assessment of these various scenarios is covered later in this chapter.

Testosterone

Testosterone is released in pulses; it has a circadian rhythm with an 8 a.m. peak and ideally should be measured at this time. Testosterone is largely bound to SHBG, with a small active free testosterone fraction. Most androgen-responsive tissues convert testosterone to dihydrotestosterone, catalysed by 5-α-reductase. Stress and exercise will reduce testosterone production. There is usually a gradual reduction in testosterone levels after age 50, but levels may remain unchanged in many men.

Oestrogens

Levels fluctuate widely depending on the timing in the cycle (see above).

Gonadotrophin-releasing hormone test

This test can distinguish between pituitary and hypothalamic disease, but this rarely has a practical indication and the test is not widely used.

One hundred micrograms of GnRH are given intravenously at 9 a.m. Blood is taken for LH and FSH at 20 and 60 min. A rise should be seen, as shown in Table 6.1.

A subnormal response to the test occurs in pituitary disease. A normal or exaggerated response occurs in hypothalamic disease.

HIRSUTISM

Hirsutism is defined as excess hair growth in women, occurring in an androgen-dependent pattern (upper lip, chin, chest, periumbilical area, inner thighs). It should be distinguished from hypertrichosis, which is an excess of long, fine, typically vellus hairs on areas such as the forehead and is not androgen-dependent.

Hirsutism occurs due to androgen excess or increased skin sensitivity to androgens. Androgens are produced from the ovaries and adrenals in equal amounts in the premenopausal woman. Box 6.1 summarizes the causes of androgen excess. An evaluation of hirsutism should take into account other features of androgen excess (Box 6.2), with a particular emphasis on a search for signs of virilization (which occurs with marked hyperandrogenism and may reflect an oncogenic source). The history should also enquire about onset and duration of hirsutism (rapid onset may be associated with an adrenal or ovarian tumour). A clinical scoring system for hirsutism (the Ferriman–Gallwey score) has been developed but is relatively insensitive in clinical practice, and a more useful assessment is the time spent each day on hair removal.

Investigation

The majority of patients will have polycystic ovary syndrome (PCOS) or idiopathic hirsutism. Investigation is aimed at detecting the minority who may have a virilizing tumour or a condition such as Cushing's syndrome that requires a different approach. Box 6.3 shows the biochemical tests that should be performed in a patient presenting with hirsutism.

If there is virilization or the androgens are high (testosterone >5 nmol/L), then ovarian and adrenal imaging (magnetic resonance imaging, MRI, or computerized tomography) is

---

Box 6.1: Causes of androgen excess

Common

- Polycystic ovary syndrome
- Idiopathic
- Increased free androgens due to low sex hormone-binding globulin (e.g. in obesity)

Infrequent

- Cushing's syndrome

Rare

- Virilizing tumours of the ovary and adrenal
- Hyperthecosis ovarii
- Congenital adrenal hyperplasia

Box 6.2: Other features of androgen excess

- Androgenic alopecia: the loss of scalp hair in an androgenic pattern in women (i.e. from the top of the head). If the hair loss is equal on the sides of the head and the top of the head, then this is diffuse idiopathic hair loss. Mild temporal recession is common in adolescence.
- Acne.
- Clitoromegaly (virilization).
- Deepening of the voice (virilization).
- Increased muscle bulk (virilization).

Box 6.3: Biochemical investigation of hirsutism

- Testosterone, sex hormone-binding globulin, androstenedione, dehydroepiandrosterone sulphate
- Luteinizing hormone, follicle-stimulating hormone, oestradiol
- 17-Hydroxyprogesterone (optional; measure at 9 a.m. in the follicular phase of the menstrual cycle; may need to proceed to a synacthen test if raised – see Ch. 5)
- A 1-mg overnight dexamethasone suppression test, 24-h urinary free cortisol or late night salivary cortisol (if signs of possible Cushing's syndrome)

Box 6.4: Treatments of hirsutism

- Mechanical removal (waxing, plucking, shaving, depilatory creams)
- Laser removal
- Electrolysis
- Eflornithine 11.5% cream
- Oestrogens
- Antiandrogens

---

required to search for tumours or hyperthecosis ovarii (an exaggerated form of PCOS). Patients with persistent hyperandrogenism and an equivocal or negative imaging study will require further evaluation with selective adrenal and ovarian vein sampling to determine the source of androgen excess, especially if a formal low-dose dexamethasone suppression test fails to demonstrate testosterone suppression.

Treatment

Hirsutism progresses with time, so reassurance is not appropriate. Treatments are listed in Box 6.4. A woman should be able to assess the severity of the hirsutism herself, as the same degree of hirsutism will have a different adverse impact on different women. Mechanical hair removal (shaving, plucking, waxing) does not worsen the hirsutism but is usually unsatisfactory. The aim is to return hair to finer vellus hair. Because hair changes slowly, any treatment will need at least 6 months to judge efficacy. If the diagnosis is PCOS, the metabolic, menstrual or fertility features may also need addressing (see p. 147 and Ch. 7).

Laser therapy is an effective treatment for facial hirsutism, but previous claims of permanent hair removal have been tempered with the recognition that hair growth recurs after a period of time. There are a number of lasers available, with no clear evidence at present to support the use of one over another, although skin colour impacts on choice. Treatment is usually given in six cycles, but the cost of this treatment (it is not routinely available on the UK National Health Service) is often prohibitive for many patients.

Electrolysis is also an effective treatment, although it is again expensive and patients may require a number of treatment sessions if their hirsutism is extensive.

Eflornithine is an irreversible inhibitor of ornithine decarboxylase, a key regulatory enzyme in hair follicle growth. It is licensed for the treatment of facial hirsutism and should be applied twice daily to affected areas. Patients should be advised to continue with mechanical hair removal and should be warned not to expect significant benefit for at least 2 months.

Oestrogens suppress ovarian androgen production and raise SHBG, thereby reducing free androgens. These are frequently prescribed in combination with an antiandrogen (Dianette: ethinyloestradiol 35 μg, cyproterone acetate 2 mg), although there is little convincing evidence that this is any more effective than combined oral contraceptive pills (OCPs) alone. A careful evaluation of risk factors for venous thrombosis, including family history, must always precede prescription of the OCP, especially with Dianette, which probably carries a slightly higher risk of venous thrombosis than third-generation OCPs. A recently available OCP preparation containing 30 μg of ethinyloestradiol and 3 mg of the antiandrogenic progestogen drospirenone (Yasmin) may also have equivalent efficacy in improving hirsutism.

Antiandrogens block the androgen receptor or block the conversion of testosterone to dihydrotestosterone. Many carry a risk of significant toxicity and are therefore reserved for patients who have failed to respond to other measures. Spironolactone can be used in a dose of 50–200 mg a day. This may increase the frequency of menses to every 2 weeks and is unsafe in pregnancy (toxicity seen in animal studies), thus ideally should be used in combination with the OCP. It may be useful in postmenopausal hirsutism when oestrogen preparations may be unsuitable. Cyproterone acetate can be started at 50 mg/day, but if it is used continuously it will cause amenorrhoea and possibly hypogonadism. It is therefore given for the first 10 days of the cycle or combined with the OCP. There is a risk of hepatotoxicity and fetotoxicity, and the patient must be counselled about this. The patient should be monitored with a haemoglobin measurement, as there is a risk of anaemia, and also should have regular liver function tests. Flutamide 125–250 mg twice daily can also be used. This has side-effects of low libido, dry skin and amenorrhoea. It is toxic in pregnancy and can cause fatal hepatotoxicity, and again the patient must be counselled carefully prior to commencing this treatment. Finasteride is a 5-α-reductase inhibitor. It is very effective and well tolerated but is very toxic to male fetuses (causing feminization), and its use is thus usually restricted to surgically sterilized or postmenopausal women.

MENSTRUAL DISTURBANCE

This can be divided into:

- amenorrhoea (no menstrual bleeding for over 6 months)
- oligomenorrhoea
- polymenorrhoea
- menorrhagia.

Polymenorrhoea and menorrhagia may be related to hypothyroidism but usually reflect dysfunctional uterine bleeding and will not be considered further here.

Primary amenorrhoea, secondary amenorrhoea and oligomenorrhoea have causes that can be subdivided into three groups.

1. Primary ovarian failure (see p. 149).
2. PCOS (see p. 147).
3. Disordered gonadotrophin secretion (hypogonadotrophic hypogonadism), which may be due to hypothalamic–pituitary disease (Ch. 1), be due to functional disease or be idiopathic. Functional (or 'hypothalamic') oligomenorrhoea or amenorrhoea may be secondary to low body weight (e.g. in anorexia nervosa), intensive exercise, psychogenic disease (e.g. stress) or significant intercurrent illness. Weight loss and exercise suppress the gonadotrophin pulsatility. As weight returns, menses will return but often after a time lag of several months. Stress and illness also affect hypothalamic control of gonadotrophins.

Clinical features

The history should cover the presence of features of oestrogen deficiency (e.g. hot flushes, vaginal dryness), galactorrhoea, the onset of menstrual disturbance, weight change, exercise and significant intercurrent illness. Examination should include a search for features of virilization and other endocrine disease.

Investigation

A pregnancy test is indicated if the history is short. Subsequent biochemical and radiological tests may depend on features elicited during the clinical evaluation of the patient but can be broadly centred on results of oestradiol and gonadotrophin measurements. Figure 6.3 provides a suggested flowchart for the evaluation of amenorrhoea and oligomenorrhoea.

Figure 6.3
Investigative approach to the evaluation of oligomenorrhoea or amenorrhoea.

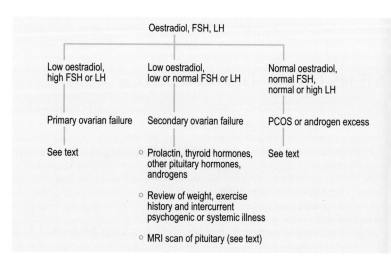

POLYCYSTIC OVARY SYNDROME

There has been some controversy about the definition of PCOS, but the Rotterdam consensus review states that PCOS is diagnosed in the presence of two out of the following three criteria, provided that other causes of polycystic ovaries are excluded (e.g. Cushing's syndrome and congenital adrenal hyperplasia):

1. clinical or biochemical features of hyperandrogenism
2. oligo-ovulation or anovulation
3. ultrasound features of PCOS.

Polycystic ovary syndrome affects up to 8% of women of reproductive age and is the commonest cause of subfertility. The ultrasound features are not diagnostic alone, as 20% of premenopausal women will have the typical appearance. In those who are asymptomatic, the appearance of polycystic ovaries on sonography does not appear to have any implications in relation to ill health, such as subfertility.

Pathophysiology

Both obese and lean women with PCOS have insulin resistance. Insulin resistance varies with menstrual pattern and is greatest in women with the most significant oligomenorrhoea. There is also a relative defect of insulin secretion, which does not improve with weight loss, in contrast to insulin resistance. Current evidence points to a selective tissue insulin resistance with preservation of insulin sensitivity in the ovary, leading to an exaggeration of the normal effects of insulin on stimulation of ovarian steroidogenesis. Insulin also acts synergistically with LH, which is secreted with increased pulse frequency to increase ovarian androgen synthesis. Adrenal androgen synthesis is also increased. Insulin action in the liver contributes further to the increased androgen activity by reduction of SHBG levels.

Clinical features

These are summarized in Box 6.5.

Box 6.5: Clinical features of polycystic ovary syndrome

- Menstrual irregularity, which often starts soon after the menarche or after a period of weight gain
- Subfertility due to anovulatory cycles
- Hirsutism and acne
- Virilization may be present but should always prompt a search for a virilizing tumour
- Recurrent miscarriages
- More than 50% of patients are obese with an increased central distribution (raised waist circumference)
- Difficulty losing weight
- A family history of premature adrenarche, polycystic ovary syndrome or type 2 diabetes may be present

Complications

With advancing age, insulin resistance and loss of insulin production may contribute to glucose intolerance and type 2 diabetes. Features of the metabolic syndrome are present in a substantial proportion of patients, and up to 15% will have diabetes in later life (compared with 2% of control subjects). Obesity and a family history of type 2 diabetes compound this risk, with up to 40% of obese subjects with PCOS developing either frank diabetes or impaired glucose tolerance. These adverse metabolic features have not yet been proven to result in premature vascular mortality, although case control studies suggest an increased prevalence of markers of cardiovascular risk such as endothelial dysfunction, reduced arterial compliance and increased carotid artery intima media thickness. Many studies have shown an adverse 'proatherogenic' lipid profile in patients with PCOS (raised triglycerides, low high-density lipoprotein cholesterol), although studies on prevalence of hypertension have been inconclusive and difficult to interpret because of the confounding influence of obesity. The presence of these adverse markers should prompt careful cardiometabolic risk assessment and management in the long-term follow-up of these patients.

Unopposed oestrogen from chronic anovulation may constitute a risk factor for endometrial hyperplasia and cancer, although there is little epidemiological evidence to support this. Nevertheless, this risk should be addressed in the clinic by therapies aimed at minimizing endometrial hyperplasia (induction of menstruation by metformin, OCP or cyclic progestogens; endometrial protection with Mirena coil).

Investigations

This is largely a clinical diagnosis. Tests are primarily performed to exclude other causes of the clinical features of this syndrome and to screen for complications.

Testosterone can be as high as the low normal male range, especially in luteal hyperthecosis, but values greater than 5 nmol/L should prompt a search for other causes (see p. 143). Androstenedione and dehydroepiandrosterone sulphate (DHEAS) may be moderately elevated and the SHBG may be low. A greater pulse frequency of LH with a normal FSH can give rise to an abnormal LH:FSH ratio. The prolactin may be modestly elevated in a minority of subjects but often responds to insulin sensitization. Patients with persistent hyperprolactinaemia should be assessed to exclude a coexisting microprolactinoma (see Ch. 1). Transvaginal ultrasound of the ovaries shows multiple small subcapsular follicles and increased central stroma. Ultrasonography will also allow assessment of endometrial thickness and will identify up to 90% of virilizing ovarian tumours. It is important to recognize that the appearance of polycystic ovaries can be seen in androgen-producing tumours, late-onset congenital adrenal hyperplasia, Cushing's syndrome and hyperprolactinaemia. Furthermore, the ovarian ultrasound may be normal. An ovarian ultrasound is not essential unless the patient is virilized or the diagnosis is not established on clinical grounds. A fasting glucose and serum lipid profile should also be measured. Screening for dyslipidaemia need not necessarily commence in young patients (<30 years), as predicted 10-year cardiovascular risk would rarely be high enough to justify lipid-lowering therapy as primary prevention.

Once the diagnosis of PCOS is established, the main desired outcome should be assessed. This could be a reduction of hirsutism, pregnancy, regular menstruation or weight loss.

Treatment

The treatment of oligomenorrhoea, infertility and metabolic factors often involves reducing insulin resistance. This may be achieved either through lifestyle measures or through medication.

Weight loss, whether achieved through diet, exercise or antiobesity medication (e.g. orlistat), is effective in improving many of the manifestations of the syndrome and is a cornerstone of management.

Metformin (500 mg three times a day) may be useful for restoration of ovulatory cycles and improving fertility, though recent evidence suggests that clomiphene is more effective (see Ch. 7). Patients should be counselled to expect gastrointestinal side-effects at the start of treatment (the starting dose should be no higher than 500 mg twice daily), which tend to ease with continued administration.

Other drugs that improve insulin sensitivity may have benefit (e.g. thiazolidinediones, cannabinoid receptor 1 antagonists), but trials to confirm this are awaited. A previous study confirmed a beneficial effect of troglitazone on a number of aspects of the syndrome, but this has since been discontinued.

Patients not desiring fertility can be prescribed the OCP to induce a regular menstrual cycle, or alternatively can be given cyclic progestogens or have a Mirena coil inserted to ensure endometrial protection.

For hirsutism treatment, see page 144.

PRIMARY OVARIAN FAILURE

Primary ovarian failure usually presents with primary or secondary amenorrhoea. The most common cause is idiopathic premature ovarian failure, followed by Turner's syndrome. The median age of the menopause in the UK is 50 years; menopause before the age of 40 is described as premature ovarian failure. Those conditions that affect ovarian development may present with primary amenorrhoea and lack of secondary sexual characteristics. Table 6.2 summarizes the causes of primary ovarian failure.

Autoimmune

Autoimmune polyendocrinopathy syndrome types 1 and 2 are described in Chapter 5 and may both be associated with premature ovarian failure. Circulating autoantibodies against the ovaries are sometimes found in premature ovarian failure, and a fifth of women will have other autoimmune disease.

Table 6.2: Causes of primary ovarian failure

Category	Details
Idiopathic	Most common cause
Autoimmune	Type 1 and type 2 autoimmune polyglandular syndrome Isolated autoimmune
Iatrogenic	Surgery, radiotherapy, chemotherapy
Genetic	Familial ovarian failure Galactosaemia Enzyme defects: P450c17 Fragile X permutations/blepharophimosis, ptosis and epicanthus inversus syndrome Follicle-stimulating hormone receptor mutation
Infection	Viral oophoritis
Gonadal dysgenesis	Turner's syndrome Perrault's syndrome 46XY gonadal dysgenesis 46XX gonadal dysgenesis

The surgical procedure of hysterectomy may damage ovarian blood supply and cause ovarian failure. Chemotherapy and radiotherapy can cause primary ovarian failure. For example, around 50% of survivors of childhood haematological malignancies will have ovarian failure, but spontaneous remission is more common in this group than with other causes. Viral oophoritis will develop in around 5% of women with mumps.

Turner's syndrome is the commonest cause of gonadal dysgenesis, but gonadal dysgenesis can occur in a 46XX karyotype in which the cause is unknown. Patients with 46XY karyotypes are at risk of malignant transformation of the gonads, and removal (usually laparoscopically) is needed. Perrault's syndrome is an autosomal recessive condition characterized by congenital deafness, short stature and gonadal dysgenesis.

Turner's syndrome

The most common karyotype is 45X0, but any X chromosomal defect can cause Turner's syndrome; occasionally, only some of the cells have the abnormal X chromosome – this is termed *mosaicism*. There is a variable phenotype, but the most consistent features are hypogonadism and short stature. The clinical features of Turner's syndrome are shown in Figure 6.4.

Management of Turner's syndrome

The principles of treatment for patients with Turner's syndrome can be broadly divided into the following categories:

- to screen for and prevent complications (e.g. aortic dissection, diabetes, thyroid dysfunction)

Dysmorphic features
- Webbed neck
- Epicanthal folds
- Broad chest, wide-spaced nipples
- Cubitus valgus
- Short fourth metacarpal

Audiology
- Otitis media
- Progressive sensorineural deafness

Cardiac
- Congenital heart disease (40%)
- Left heart lesions cause susceptibility to infective endocarditis
- Bicuspid aortic valve
- Coarctation of aorta (10%)
- Aortic dissection

Hepatic
- Raised liver enzymes
- Fatty infiltration and fibrosis

Renal
- Congenital anomalies (increased nine fold)

Metabolic
- Ischaemic heart disease (increased nine fold)
- Hypertension (risk tripled)
- Type 2 diabetes (2–4 times the risk)
- Insulin resistance (50%)
- Hyperlipididaemia

Neurological/psychological
- Reduced visuospacial ability
- Reduced motor coordination
- Reduced ability to befriend
- Reduced sexual relationships

Thyroid
- 50% positive antibodies
- Hypo- and hyperthyroidism

Skeletal
- Short stature
- Osteoporosis
- Lymphoedema

Intestinal
- Intestinal telangectasia
- Inflammatory bowel disease (2–3 times the risk)

Gonadal dysgenesis
- Primary amenorrhoea
- Delayed puberty
- Streak ovaries
- Spontaneous puberty (16%) (40% in mosaics)
- Spontaneous pregnancy (5%)
- 40% of conceptions result in non-viable pregnancies

Cancer
- Gonadoblastoma in those with XY mosaicism –prophylactic gonadectomy needed

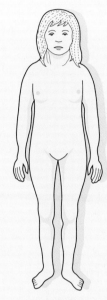

Overall
Tripled increase in mortality

Figure 6.4
Features of Turner's syndrome.

- to achieve optimum symptom control (e.g. best final height, induction of puberty; see Ch. 2)
- to facilitate pregnancy by ovum donation (see Ch. 7).

Adult patients with Turner's syndrome have an increased risk of a number of complications in the long term (Fig. 6.4), and continued follow-up is therefore mandatory.

Oestrogen replacement therapy should be started in low doses and built up gradually to allow normal development of secondary sexual characteristics. Introduction of oestrogen replacement should not be too early because of potential negative consequences on optimal final height, but should not be unduly delayed to ensure maximization of uterine development, which has implications for future pregnancy. On average, oestrogen therapy is commenced at the age of 13 years. Pelvic ultrasonography may be used to assess uterine development. In adult practice, oestrogen may be given as the OCP or hormone replacement therapy (HRT), although trials are currently examining the effects of these alternatives on outcome. Trials are also examining the effects of oxandrolone on height.

The possibility of future pregnancy with ovum donation should be discussed. If presentation is before epiphyseal fusion, then growth hormone treatment should be offered.

An echocardiogram should be performed every 3 years but repeated annually if abnormal. If the aortic root is dilated, an MRI scan may provide more detailed assessment. An audiogram every 3 years detects hearing loss, and bone mineral density should be measured every 3 years. Renal ultrasonography detects renal tract abnormalities.

In view of the excess cardiovascular risk, annual blood pressure measurements should be made (beta blockers or calcium antagonists may be used for therapy). In addition, annual fasting glucose and lipids, thyroid function tests, urea and electrolytes and liver function tests should be done.

Contact details for Turner's syndrome support groups should be supplied.

Clinical features of primary ovarian failure

These will depend on the timing of the failure; gonadal dysgenesis usually results in primary amenorrhoea and lack of secondary sexual characteristics, whereas premature ovarian failure will result in secondary amenorrhoea.

Investigations

- Raised FSH and LH, low oestrogen (FSH should be measured at intervals several weeks apart, as transient ovarian failure can occur).
- Chromosomal analysis.
- Ovarian antibodies will be found only in a small proportion.
- Pelvic ultrasound is not usually helpful (it can help to identify gonads prior to removal in XY gonadal dysgenesis).

Treatment

Hormone replacement is needed to treat the oestrogen deficiency and to prevent osteoporosis. Ideal replacement is suboptimal in premenopausal women, as the oral contraceptive gives supraphysiological replacement for 3 out of 4 weeks and most HRTs are formulated for replacement in older women. Ovum donation is usually required for fertility, although rarely spontaneous ovulation can occur. Bone mineral density should be measured at baseline and during follow-up by dual energy x-ray absorptiometry scan.

MALE HYPOGONADISM

Male hypogonadism can be divided into primary and secondary hypogonadism, according to whether the gonadotrophins are, respectively, elevated or not in the presence of a low testosterone level. A number of causes are recognized (Box 6.6).

Box 6.6: Causes of male hypogonadism

Primary failure

- Surgical castration
- Trauma or torsion of testes
- Cryptorchidism (early orchidopexy helps)
- Drug or surgical treatment for prostatic and penile cancer
- Testicular artery damage (e.g. mistakenly at vasectomy)
- Varicocoele
- Infections (viral, e.g. 25% with mumps orchitis, granulomatous)
- Infiltration (e.g. sarcoidosis)
- Irradiation
- Autoimmune
- Drugs (e.g. cyproterone, spironolactone)
- Chromosomal abnormalities (e.g. Klinefelter's syndrome, XYY syndrome, XX male syndrome, gonadal dysgenesis)
- Systemic illness (e.g. paraplegia, renal failure, cirrhosis)

Secondary failure

Pituitary disease

- Tumours such as non-functioning adenomas
- Hyperprolactinaemia
- Cushing's syndrome (any aetiology)
- Surgery, irradiation, infarction, infiltration

Hypothalamic disease

- Craniopharyngioma
- Constitutional delay
- Kallmann's syndrome
- Prader–Willi syndrome
- Specific luteinizing hormone deficiency
- Secondary disorders of gonadotrophin-releasing hormone secretion (e.g. drug abuse, malnutrition)
- Laurence–Moon–Biedl syndrome
- Pasqualini syndrome

Evaluation should include a careful history to determine previous cryptorchidism, childhood mumps or testicular surgery and previous chemoradiotherapy, and a systemic enquiry in addition to a search for symptoms related to hypogonadism per se. Patients should be asked if they have previously fathered children.

Klinefelter's syndrome

Klinefelter's syndrome (47XXY karyotype) is probably the commonest cause of primary hypogonadism, occurring in as many as one in 1000 births, although many will go unnoticed and the condition is usually unsuspected prepubertally. There is a wide phenotypic spectrum ranging from normal virilization to feminization; the clinical features are illustrated in Figure 6.5. FSH levels are very high with normal to high LH (testosterone replacement will not normalize these). Testosterone levels are highest in the late teens and then fall; oestradiol may be raised. A full range of karyotypes may occur,

Figure 6.5
Features of Klinefelter's syndrome.

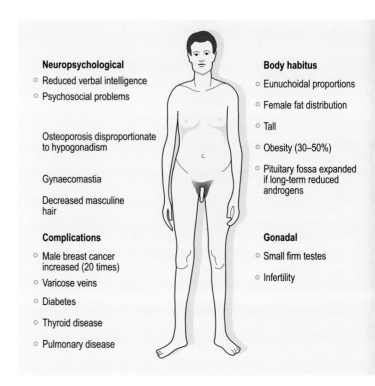

Neuropsychological
- Reduced verbal intelligence
- Psychosocial problems

Osteoporosis disproportionate to hypogonadism

Gynaecomastia

Decreased masculine hair

Complications
- Male breast cancer increased (20 times)
- Varicose veins
- Diabetes
- Thyroid disease
- Pulmonary disease

Body habitus
- Eunuchoidal proportions
- Female fat distribution
- Tall
- Obesity (30–50%)
- Pituitary fossa expanded if long-term reduced androgens

Gonadal
- Small firm testes
- Infertility

with some phenotypic consequences (e.g. 46XY/47XXY mosaics may be less affected and retain fertility while 48XXYY patients are usually taller with lower IQ).

Kallmann's syndrome

This is an isolated gonadotrophin deficiency often but not invariably associated with anosmia or hyposmia (due to failure of olfactory lobe development). Kallmann's syndrome usually occurs sporadically but can be inherited in an autosomal dominant, autosomal recessive or X-linked manner. Until recently, defects in the KAL-1 gene were the only recognized molecular cause of this condition, although mutations in the fibroblast growth factor receptor-1 (FGFR-1) gene have now been described in a number of families. The phenotypic expression of the disease varies both between and within families. In addition to hypogonadism and olfactory dysfunction, other manifestations include cleft palate, colour blindness, sensorineural deafness, renal abnormalities, cryptorchidism, micropenis and bimanual synkinesis ('mirror movements').

Clinical features of male hypogonadism

If hypogonadism occurs prepubertally, the clinical features may include microphallus, delayed epiphyseal closure leading to eunuchoidal proportions (the span exceeding the vertical height by >5 cm), cryptorchidism with potential for malignant change, and impaired laryngeal growth leading to a high-pitched voice.

If hypogonadism occurs either pre- or postpubertally, then reduced libido and impotence may occur. Infertility can occur, as testosterone is needed for spermatogenesis. Body hair loss is variable in hypogonadism, and there may be a lack of masculine hair (facial hair, chest and back hair, upwards extension of pubic hair and change to vellus hair on the scalp). Gynaecomastia may be present, and osteoporosis may occur with reduced upper body musculature and a thin skin.

Investigations

A testosterone level should be measured at 8–9 a.m., as afternoon samples may be misleadingly low. SHBG is helpful to estimate the bioavailable testosterone; alternatively, free testosterone is available in some laboratories and may be particularly useful if the result is borderline low (such as in ageing men). LH and FSH should be measured, and prolactin measured if they are normal or low. If the gonadotrophins are high, a chromosomal analysis should be performed. Further investigations (e.g. pituitary MRI scan) will depend on other findings.

Treatment

Treatment is by androgen replacement (see p. 159) unless fertility is desired, in which case gonadotrophin therapy (or pulsatile GnRH therapy in hypothalamic disease) may be tried in secondary hypogonadism.

GYNAECOMASTIA

This is benign hyperplasia of the breast tissue in men. Clinically, it is important to distinguish between true gynaecomastia and adiposity, which can be difficult. Testosterone inhibits the development of the breast, whereas oestrogens stimulate development. A relative excess of oestrogens may be due to overproduction or administration of oestrogens, underproduction of androgens or an altered androgen:oestrogen ratio.

Physiological causes

Gynaecomastia can occur in the newborn, at puberty or in advancing age. Around 50% of 14-year-old boys will have gynaecomastia, which usually disappears spontaneously. Pathological causes of gynaecomastia are shown in Box 6.7.

Clinical features

The history and examination will largely determine which investigations to perform.

Measurement of testosterone, LH, FSH, SHBG and oestradiol will reveal if excess oestrogen or insufficient androgen is causal. It is usual to measure the prolactin, although   155

Box 6.7: Pathological causes of gynaecomastia

- Idiopathic
- Drugs:
  —oestrogens (e.g. for prostate cancer treatment or inadvertent exposure such as vaginal oestrogens from a partner)
  —antiandrogens (e.g. spironolactone, cimetidine, cyproterone)
  —cytotoxic drugs
  —recreational drugs (cannabis)
- Increased production of oestrogens or human chorionic gonadotrophin:
  —testicular, adrenal or lung tumours
- Deficient androgen production:
  —Klinefelter syndrome
  —primary testicular failure
  —androgen resistance syndromes
  —hypopituitarism
  —non-virilizing congenital adrenal hyperplasia
- Altered oestrogen:testosterone ratio:
  —liver disease (reduced oestrogen clearance)
  —renal disease
  —thyrotoxicosis (elevated sex hormone-binding globulin causes a relative lack of free testosterone)
  —Cushing's syndrome
  —acromegaly
  —starvation and refeeding

---

it is a misconception that hyperprolactinaemia causes gynaecomastia. Thyroid, renal and liver function tests should be done, as should a karyotype to detect Klinefelter syndrome. Testicular (or occasionally lung) tumours may produce hCG or α-fetoprotein, so these should be measured.

The most common reasons for gynaecomastia are drugs and chronic disease. Other patients will usually have idiopathic gynaecomastia.

Treatment

The underlying cause should be addressed whenever possible. Patients with physiological pubertal gynaecomastia should be reassured that it will probably resolve in 1–2 years. Some idiopathic gynaecomastia will also resolve. Drug treatment is often unsuccessful, but anastrazole and tamoxifen have both been used. Tamoxifen may be useful to prevent gynaecomastia during antiandrogen treatment for prostatic cancer. Surgical correction of gynaecomastia may be needed in resistant or severe cases or in milder cases when psychological stress is significant.

ERECTILE DYSFUNCTION

Erectile dysfunction is the inability to attain a penile erection sufficient for sexual intercourse. This can occur in around 50% of men over the age of 40 years. A number of causes are described (Table 6.3).

Table 6.3: Causes of erectile dysfunction

Cause	Details
Psychological	–
Organic	
Anatomical	Surgery or trauma to the pelvic area, blood supply or spinal cord
Vascular	Coronary artery disease, diabetes
Neurogenic	Alzheimer disease, cerebral vascular accidents, Parkinson disease, multiple sclerosis, spina bifida
Hormonal	Testosterone deficiency, but libido is more affected by sex hormone anomalies than erectile function
Drug-related	See text
Chronic disease	Renal or hepatic failure, arthritis, pulmonary disease
Lifestyle	Smoking, alcohol, obesity

Drug-related causes can be divided into four main groups. Antiandrogens such as cyproterone, spironolactone, cimetidine and digoxin comprise one group. Antihypertensives such as thiazides, beta blockers and angiotensin-converting enzyme inhibitors may be implicated in the aetiology of erectile dysfunction; however, they are commonly prescribed in vascular disease, so it may be difficult to know whether the relationship is causal. This is also the case for lipid-lowering drugs such as statins and fibrates. Centrally acting drugs such as tricyclic antidepressant drugs, methyldopa, clonidine and carbamazepine can all cause erectile dysfunction.

Erectile dysfunction can be considered as an early marker of vascular disease in some disorders (e.g. diabetes and coronary artery disease). The penile arteries are a third of the diameter of the coronary arteries and are thus susceptible to atherosclerosis. The development of erectile dysfunction in men with diabetes should prompt a full review of risk factors for vascular disease.

Treatment of erectile dysfunction

An underlying cause should be sought and treated whenever possible, and this may be sufficient to restore potency on its own (e.g. dopamine agonist treatment of hyperprolactinaemia). In patients who do not respond to such measures or when no underlying cause can be found, a stepwise approach to management should be considered. First-line drug treatment is usually with phosphodiesterase type V inhibitors (sildenafil, tadalafil, vardenafil), and sublingual apomorphine can also be used. Intracavernosal or urethral alprostadil may be successful, whereas other patients may prefer a vacuum tumescence device. Penile implants using prostheses or other mechanical devices may be used. Psychosexual therapy for couples may be helpful.

OESTROGEN REPLACEMENT THERAPY

Postmenopausal therapy

Hormone replacement therapy in the form of oestrogens and progestogens is used for controlling menopausal symptoms. It has previously been used for osteoporosis prevention and treatment and to prevent cardiovascular disease and dementia. It is now indicated only for short-term use (<5 years) for menopausal symptoms. The menopause causes physiological symptoms such as hot flushes, night sweats and mood disturbance. Low oestrogen levels may also have adverse effects on the genitourinary tract, such as atrophic vaginitis, stress incontinence and urinary tract infections.

The optimum HRT combination, route of administration and dose are not known. HRT may be given orally, subcutaneously, transdermally or intranasally. Local oestrogens can successfully treat the genitourinary symptoms, in the form of intravaginal tablets or rings, creams and gels. HRT preparations may include natural oestrogens such as oestradiol, oestrone and oestriol or synthetic oestrogens such as ethinyloestradiol and mestranol; naturally occurring oestrogens have a better profile for HRT. Transdermal oestradiol results in 10-fold lower circulating oestrone sulphate than oral preparations. Oral oestrogen therapy increases SHBG to a greater extent than that given by alternative routes, which may alter bioavailability. Patients on systemic HRT with an intact uterus require oestrogens plus progestogens to reduce the risk of endometrial cancer. The progestogens can either be given continually or for the last 12–14 days of the cycle.

Hormone replacement therapy increases the risk of thromboembolic disease; this may not be the case for transdermal oestrogen, although there is insufficient evidence to be certain. HRT increases the risk of breast cancer (1.5–6 extra cases per 1000 women in 5 years); this risk is greater for oestrogens combined with progestogens, and a longer duration of use increases the risk. HRT prevents bone loss and fractures but is no longer used solely for this purpose, as there are other effective alternatives that have fewer adverse effects. Evidence is conflicting on the cardiovascular effects of HRT. Some observational studies have shown trends towards a protective effect; however, a large primary prevention trial (Women's Health Initiative) showed an increased risk of acute myocardial infarction. This was a study of equine oestrogen and medroxyprogesterone or oestrogen alone, and it has been suggested that a continuous regimen rather than a cyclic regimen caused the adverse outcomes. There is also an increased risk of stroke and gall bladder disease, and HRT does not reduce the risk of dementia. There is possibly a reduced risk of colon cancer and possibly an increased risk of ovarian cancer; however, the Women's Health Initiative study did not confirm either of these suggestions.

Tibolone is a synthetic steroid. Tibolone and the metabolites of tibolone have oestrogenic, progestogenic and androgenic properties. Tibolone largely results in a progestogenic effect in the endometrium such that other progestogens are not required and cyclic bleeding does not occur. This should not be used within 12 months of the last menstrual period or it may cause irregular bleeding. Tibolone also increases the risk of breast cancer, but there is insufficient evidence to know if it predisposes to thromboembolic disease.

Selective oestrogen receptor modulators such as raloxifene have selective oestrogenic and antioestrogenic effects in different tissues. Raloxifene has oestrogen agonist effects on the bone and on lipids and oestrogen antagonist effects on the breast and the endometrium. Raloxifene may reduce the risk of vertebral fractures, but there is an increased risk of venous thromboembolism and the symptoms of hot flushes and vaginal dryness may be worsened.

Premenopausal hormone replacement therapy

Hypogonadism due to conditions such as Turner's syndrome will require HRT, which should be initiated at a physiological age and continued until the usual age of menopause, although a minority of patients may enter puberty spontaneously. HRT in this situation should allow the development of secondary sexual characteristics at an appropriate time, have psychosocial advantages, allow normal uterine development and result in normal bone mineral density. Oestrogen therapy should be started at a low dose and gradually increased to allow this development. Both the combined OCP and 'menopausal' HRT are used in this situation, but neither is ideal. Transdermal oestrogens with oral progestogens may be a preferred regimen.

ANDROGEN REPLACEMENT THERAPY

Testosterone therapy is used to treat hypogonadal men and, more recently, used to treat androgen deficiency in the ageing male (ADAM) and as an adjunct in treating menopausal symptoms in women. Testosterone is available in various forms. Testosterone propionate is injected every 2–3 weeks and will peak 2–5 days postinjection and fall to basal levels at 2 weeks; it thus has very variable blood levels but is inexpensive. Transdermal testosterone can be given in the form of patches and gels, which give consistent plasma levels and are easy to apply. Subcutaneous implants are available that give constant levels for 4–5 months; however, the newer 3-monthly intramuscular injection of testosterone undecanoate has largely superseded these. Buccal testosterone is available as is oral testosterone, although the latter is rarely used due to poor bioavailability.

Testosterone increases lean mass, reduces fat mass, increases upper and lower body strength, increases libido and sex function, and improves mood. It also has an effect on cognitive function, improving spatial ability and verbal memory. It increases bone mineral density and restores haemoglobin in anaemia associated with hypogonadism.

As cardiovascular disease is more prevalent in men, testosterone has been suggested as a risk factor. Studies have not shown an increased risk of cardiovascular disease in testosterone-treated men, and some have shown benefits, although large-scale studies are needed to confirm or refute this.

The changes on lipid profile in studies have included a lowering of the high-density lipoprotein cholesterol and also a lowering of the low-density lipoprotein cholesterol, with probably an overall neutral effect.

Testosterone increases erythropoiesis, probably to a greater extent with injections than with transdermal delivery. Any resulting polycythaemia may have a deleterious effect on vascular disease; however, there is no evidence of an increased risk of thromboembolic disease.

Prostatic volume increases with testosterone treatment, but it is unusual for this to result in a worsening of prostatic symptoms such as difficulty voiding urine. However, there is a potential risk for this in benign prostatic hypertrophy. Moreover, testosterone therapy may cause growth of a prostatic cancer, and occult prostatic cancers are relatively common. Prior to commencing testosterone therapy, a prostate-specific antigen (PSA) should be measured and a digital rectal examination performed to detect any occult prostatic cancers. If either of these tests is abnormal, a prostatic biopsy should be performed. A biopsy should also be performed if the digital rectal examination becomes abnormal or the PSA rises.

Oral testosterone is associated with hepatotoxicity and both benign and malignant tumours, whereas other forms of testosterone do not have these effects and are therefore preferred.

There may be a development or a worsening of sleep apnoea with testosterone treatment, which is thought to be an effect on the central nervous system rather than on the airway. Testosterone treatment will reduce spermatogenesis by reducing gonadotrophin levels, and men should be warned of this. Breast tenderness, fluid retention, acne and increased hair growth may occur.

There is a progressive decline in testosterone with ageing in men, and there may be features exhibited such as reduced sexual function, reduced muscle strength, osteoporosis and altered lean:fat ratios. Hypogonadism occurring in this setting is termed *ADAM* or *late-onset hypogonadism.* Such men may have a low normal or a slightly decreased testosterone. Given the significant disadvantages of testosterone therapy in addition to the advantages, treatment is best confined to those with a mildly low testosterone with symptoms and signs of androgen deficiency and those with significantly decreased testosterone.

Once testosterone therapy is commenced, the patient should be monitored at least annually with a PSA measurement, a digital rectal examination, a haematocrit and haemoglobin measurement, and a testosterone level. If there is a good therapeutic effect, the testosterone can remain in the lower half of the normal range, but if not the dose may need to be increased or transdermal preparations switched to injected preparations. Generally, the testosterone level should not be supraphysiological.

Androgen replacement in women improves bone density, libido and body composition. There may be some adverse features, such as hirsutism, but it is relatively well tolerated. The transdermal route is the optimal route of delivery, but large-scale trials are needed to assess safety.

Androgen replacement in the young man

Hypogonadism may present with failure to enter puberty. Androgen therapy should be timed so that it is started early enough to prevent psychosocial problems but not too early to reduce final height, and is usually started at between 14 and 16 years. Testosterone therapy should be started at a low dose and gradually increased at around 6-monthly intervals. This therapy will not restore fertility or increase testicular development. In primary gonadal failure, referral should be for assisted reproduction if fertility is desired. In hypogonadotrophic hypogonadism, testicular development and fertility can be improved with gonadotrophin therapy using hCG and human menopausal gonadotrophin (see Ch. 7). Pulsatile LHRH therapy can also be used for hypothalamic disease (e.g. Kallmann's syndrome). These two therapies can also be used if fertility is not immediately required to increase testicular volume and improve the chances of subsequent fertility.

Further reading

Anderson GL et al. 2004 Effects of conjugated equine oestrogen in postmenopausal women with hysterectomy: the Women's Health Initiative randomised controlled trial. JAMA 291: 1701–1712

Conway G 2000 Premature ovarian failure: its investigation and treatment. CME Bull Endocrinol Diabetes 3: 18–22

Conway G 2002 The impact and management of Turner's syndrome in adult life. Best Pract Res Clin Endocrinol Metab 16: 243–246

Davies SR, Dinatale I, Rivera-Woll L 2005 Post-menopausal hormone replacement therapy: from monkey glands to transdermal patches. J Endocrinol 185: 207–222

Rhoden EL, Morgentaler A 2004 Medical progress: risks of testosterone replacement therapy and recommendations for monitoring. New Engl J Med 350: 482–492

Tsilchorozidou T, Overton C, Conway G 2004 The pathophysiology of polycystic ovary syndrome. Clin Endocrinol 60: 1–17

SELF-ASSESSMENT

Patient 1

A 21-year-old lady is referred to you with a history of amenorrhoea and hirsutism.

Questions
1. What features would you elicit in the history and examination?
2. Which biochemical tests would you request?

Answers
1. Key features to elicit in the history would include the duration and rate of onset of the hirsutism and amenorrhoea. The previous menstrual history should be established, including timing of the menarche and any prior oligomenorrhoea. The history should also cover other symptoms of hyperandrogenism (such as scalp hair loss and acne), drug history (e.g. danazol) and family history (e.g. of type 2 diabetes or PCOS). The examination should seek to confirm the presence of hirsutism (as opposed to hypertrichosis) and describe its extent. Acanthosis nigricans may be present in the axillae or over the nape of the neck. Features of virilization (frontal balding, deepened voice, increased muscle bulk or clitoromegaly) should be looked for, as should signs of other endocrinopathies such as Cushing's syndrome or acromegaly.
2. A serum testosterone is the most important test, as levels greater than 5 nmol/L should prompt further investigations to exclude androgen-secreting tumours. Other tests that may be helpful include a 9 a.m. 17-hydroxyprogesterone level, androstenedione, DHEAS, SHBG, LH and FSH. Screening for Cushing's syndrome or acromegaly may be appropriate if these conditions are suspected clinically.

The history of amenorrhoea is short (6 months), and the patient had a normal menstrual cycle prior to this. Hirsutism is confirmed on examination, and she has some features of virilization (frontal balding and deepening of the voice). The testosterone is elevated at 22 nmol/L.

Question
3. What further investigations are indicated?

Answer
3. She needs urgent imaging of the ovaries and adrenal glands, as the testosterone level is strongly supportive of an androgen-secreting tumour.

A transvaginal ultrasound scan confirmed a large 10×8 cm left ovarian tumour. The patient underwent oophorectomy, with the histology demonstrating a Sertoli–Leydig cell tumour.

Patient 2

A 29-year-old gentleman is referred from the fertility department having been found to have evidence of hypogonadotrophic hypogonadism (testosterone 1.1 nmol/L, LH undetectable, FSH 0.6 U/L [normal range 1.4–18.1 U/L]).

Question
1. What questions would you ask in the history?

Answer
1. The history should include a search for symptoms of androgen deficiency, such as reduced libido, impotence and reduced frequency of shaving; drug abuse (e.g. anabolic steroids); anosmia or hyposmia; pubertal history; previous fertility; family history (of anosmia or hypogonadism); galactorrhoea; headaches; visual disturbance; and features of other endocrine disease (e.g. Cushing's syndrome or hypopituitarism).

On direct questioning, it emerges that the patient has never shaved in his life and had been treated short term with testosterone for delayed puberty. He denies anosmia, but a maternal uncle was known to have a poor sense of smell and had never fathered children, and his maternal great-uncle had needed to adopt children. Examination shows him to be markedly undermasculinized, with a micropenis, empty scrotal sac, gynaecomastia and absent secondary sexual characteristics. Neurological assessment shows subtle features of bimanual synkinesis (mirror movements).

Questions
2. What is the diagnosis?
3. How could this be confirmed?

Answers
2. The diagnosis is likely to be Kallmann's syndrome, and the family history supports an X-linked or possibly autosomal dominant inheritance. Although many patients with Kallmann's syndrome have anosmia, the phenotype is variable and its absence does not preclude the diagnosis. Mirror movements are supportive of this and may be a particular feature of the X-linked form, although they are no longer considered pathognomonic for this.
3. An MRI scan of the brain would show a normal pituitary gland and hypothalamus, but the olfactory bulbs may be absent or hypoplastic. The remainder of the pituitary function will be normal. KAL-1 gene defects can be looked for by fluorescent in situ hybridization analysis (for deletions) or sequencing but account for only a small proportion of Kallmann's cases. Defects in the FGFR-1 gene have recently emerged as an important cause of this condition.

An MRI scan of the abdomen and pelvis confirms the underdeveloped penis and scrotum and shows minimal testicular tissue only at the level of the external ring (Fig. 6.6a), an absent prostate and seminal vesicles.

Figure 6.6
Coronal magnetic resonance imaging scan of the pelvis, showing testicular development and descent. Arrows show testicular tissue **(a)** pretreatment and **(b)** 6 months post-treatment.

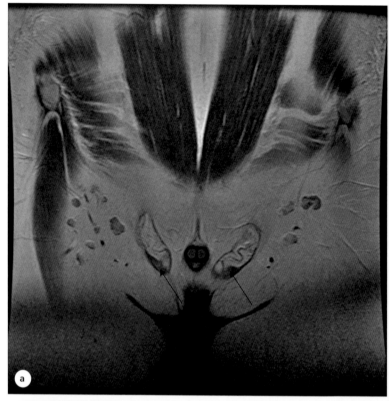

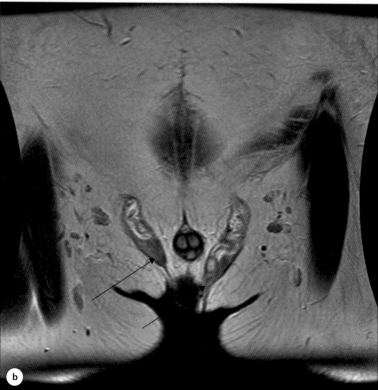

Question

4. How should this patient be treated?

Answer

4. In view of his desire for fertility, he should be treated with gonadotrophin therapy or pulsatile subcutaneous GnRH therapy.

The patient was treated with hCG 2000 U thrice weekly, which induced a significant rise in testosterone (7 nmol/L), allowing introduction of human menopausal gonadotrophin (1:1 ratio of FSH:LH). A repeat MRI scan showed development of prostatic tissue and seminal vesicles, bilateral testicular development and descent of the left testis into the scrotal sac (Fig. 6.6b).

Table 7.2: Classification of secondary amenorrhoea

Class	Cause(s)
Uterine causes	Asherman syndrome
Cervical causes	Stenosis from previous surgery, menopause, cervical lesion
Hypothalamic causes (hypogonadotrophic hypogonadism)	Weight loss Exercise Chronic illness Psychological stress Idiopathic
Pituitary causes	Hyperprolactinaemia Hypopituitarism Sheehan's syndrome
Causes of hypothalamic/pituitary damage (hypogonadism)	Tumours Cranial irradiation Head injuries Sarcoidosis Tuberculosis
Systemic causes	Chronic debilitating illness Weight loss Endocrine disorders
Chromosomal	Turner's mosaics or structural anomalies and microdeletions of second X chromosome

Tubal factors

These account for 14% of cases of infertility. Pelvic infections (pelvic inflammatory disease, PID), most commonly caused by *Chlamydia trachomatis*, result in severe tubal damage in:

- 10–30% of women after a first attack
- 30–60% after a second
- 50–90% after a third.

Chlamydial PID is often clinically 'silent' until severe pelvic adhesions and damage are identified during infertility investigations. The intrauterine contraceptive device (IUCD) may increase the risk of developing clinical PID by 50–100%, and this form of PID is often severe. Of all the different types, the progestogen-releasing IUCD (Mirena IUS) may minimize the risk of infection through its effect on cervical mucus. Because suction and medical termination of pregnancy are associated with a 5% risk of retained products of conception and hence pelvic infection, it is prudent to offer antibiotic prophylaxis to these women.

Cervical mucus factor

Around the time of ovulation, cervical mucus becomes both watery and stretchy due to the predominance of oestrogen and the lack of progesterone. At ovulation, the stretching of the mucus, known as spinnbarkeit, should be at least 8 cm. A history of previous cervical surgery should be sought and testing for chlamydial infection should be undertaken when satisfactory mucus is not seen.

Male factors

Male factors alone may be responsible in 30% and contributory in a further 20% of subfertile couples. One of the central problems in male infertility is the difficulty in identifying genuine rather than presumptive aetiological factors.

INVESTIGATION OF THE INFERTILE COUPLE

It is very important to evaluate both the female and the male partner, as a diagnosis of infertility can be made only on the basis of the results of assessments of both partners. Some barriers to pregnancy are easily identifiable, such as azoospermia, bilateral tubal obstruction or amenorrhoea. In most cases, however, the situation is less clear. A standard infertility evaluation consists of a series of tests that, despite historical roots, have had little scientific validation in distinguishing between fertile and infertile couples. When infertility evaluation identifies factors that are thought to be associated with infertility but are not absolute barriers to pregnancy, then we should counsel the couple emphasizing the gaps in our knowledge about aetiology, treatment and outcome.

Evaluation of female infertility

Particular attention needs to be paid to the reproductive history, such as previous pregnancies and their outcomes, including terminations of pregnancy. Additionally, relevant past and current gynaecological history, including characteristics of the menstrual cycle, sexually transmitted infections and information on medical/surgical illnesses, drug use/misuse and family history should be obtained. Couples also need to be questioned about their sexual activity, such as frequency and timing of sexual intercourse or sexually related problems, including loss of libido, dyspareunia and erectile or ejaculatory problems.

The general physical examination is important (Box 7.1).[3] Women who have a normal body mass index (BMI; 20–25 kg/m^2) are more likely to conceive and to have a normal pregnancy than those who are outside the normal range (Fig. 7.2).[4] Women who are underweight become anovulatory and amenorrhoeic. It is usually easy to induce ovulation in underweight women, who may then conceive readily, but these pregnancies are more likely to miscarry or result in the premature delivery of growth-restricted babies.[5] Obesity is the more common problem in western society. Not only does obesity reduce fertility, but it also increases the risk of miscarriage, gestational diabetes, hypertension, thromboembolic disease and complicated operative delivery.[6] These women should be advised to reduce their BMI to less than 30 kg/m^2 before starting any treatment. Without doubt, weight loss improves overall reproductive function,

Box 7.1: General history and examination of the female partner

History

- Previous contraception and any problems (e.g. lost coil)
- Previous pregnancies and outcome
- Medical history (pelvic infection, Crohn disease)
- Surgical history (ovarian cyst, appendectomy)
- Gynaecological history (cone biopsy, cervical smear history)
- Current medical illness
- Drug history: prescribed and misuse
- Diet
- Smoking and alcohol consumption
- Galactorrhoea
- Hirsutism
- Menstrual regularity and menorrhagia
- Dysmenorrhoea
- Intermenstrual or postcoital bleeding
- Preovulatory cervical mucus recognition
- Coital frequency and timing

Examination

- Signs of endocrine disease:
  —acne, hirsutism, balding
  —acanthosis nigricans
  —virilization
  —visual field defects
  —goitre, signs of thyroid disease
- Body mass index
- Blood pressure
- Urinalysis
- Breast examination: lumps, galactorrhoea
- Abdominal examination: masses, striae, abnormal hair growth
- Pelvic examination: clitoral appearance, evidence of cervical and vaginal endometriosis, uterine and adnexal features

(After Cahill and Wardle 2002,[3] with permission.)

Figure 7.2
Likelihood of spontaneous miscarriage and pregnancy following infertility treatment, analysed by body mass index. *95% confidence intervals do not cross unity. (After Wang et al. 2000,[4] with permission.)

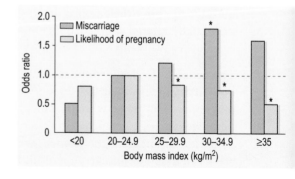

particularly in women with polycystic ovary syndrome (PCOS).[7] A pelvic examination should be performed; endometriosis is suggested by the presence of nodules in the vagina, thickening of the posterior fornix, and tenderness and limited mobility of the pelvic organs.

Signs of hyperandrogenism (acne, hirsutism, balding) are suggestive of PCOS, although biochemical screening helps to differentiate other causes of androgen excess. A testosterone level less than 5 nmol/L excludes other causes of hyperandrogenism in the majority of patients. Hirsutism can be graded according to the Ferriman–Gallwey scoring system, although the complexity of this system means that it is rarely used in clinical practice and is generally confined to research studies. It is important to distinguish between hyperandrogenism and virilization (Box 7.2). Virilization suggests a more profound disturbance of androgen secretion than usually seen with PCOS and indicates a need to exclude androgen-secreting tumours, congenital adrenal hyperplasia and Cushing's syndrome. Acanthosis nigricans is a sign of profound insulin resistance and is usually visible as hyperpigmented thickening of the skin folds of the axilla and neck. It is associated with PCOS and obesity (also Cushing's syndrome and other disorders of insulin resistance). Amenorrhoeic women may have hyperprolactinaemia with or without galactorrhoea, hence it is important to measure serum prolactin levels whether this sign is present or not. If there is suspicion of a pituitary tumour, the woman's visual fields should be checked. Thyroid disease is common, and the thyroid gland should be palpated and signs of hypothyroidism or hyperthyroidism elicited.

Evaluation of male infertility

It is important to enquire about any children from previous relationships, and to search for a history of surgery or trauma to the testes, orchitis and exposure to toxins (such as paints) or irradiation.

General examination should again include an assessment of BMI, blood pressure and secondary sexual characteristics (Box 7.3). BMI is traditionally used as an indicator of overall obesity. Men who are significantly overweight might be expected to have fertility problems as, unlike the situation in women, in men there is an inverse relationship between serum testosterone levels and visceral fat mass. Increased central obesity in men is associated with relative hypogonadism. Obesity itself is one of the several conditions

---

Box 7.2: Hyperandrogenism versus virilization

Hyperandrogenism

- Acne
- Hirsutism
- Male pattern balding

Virilization

- Acne
- Hirsutism
- Male pattern balding
- Increased muscle mass
- Deep voice
- Clitoromegaly
- Breast atrophy

Box 7.3: History and examination of the male partner

History

- Occupation (exposure to excessive heat or toxins)
- Medical history (mumps, venereal disease)
- Surgical history (orchidopexy, inguinal hernia repair, vasectomy)
- Current medical illness
- Drug history: prescribed and misuse
- Smoking and alcohol consumption
- Erectile or ejaculatory difficulty

Examination

- General: weight, height, blood pressure
- Secondary sexual characteristics
- Muscle bulk
- Signs of endocrine disease
- Gynaecomastia
- Abdominal examination: masses, hernia, scars, liver
- Genital examination: if sexual dysfunction or abnormal semen analysis

(After Cahill and Wardle 2002,[3] with permission.)

that can result in a low sex hormone-binding globulin level and is also the most common cause of insulin resistance. As a result, total testosterone is frequently low, but the free testosterone is normal, suggesting that this is not a true clinical hypogonadism. Therefore most obese men are able to reproduce normally, provided that there is no physical impediment to intercourse.

The underlying mechanisms responsible for the reduced testosterone levels in obese men are unknown. The reduction in free testosterone seen in massive obesity is not accompanied by a reciprocal increase in luteinizing hormone (LH), suggesting a form of hypogonadotrophic hypogonadism. One hypothesis postulated for the decreased free testosterone in massively obese individuals is functional alterations at the hypothalamic–pituitary level characterized by decreased amplitude of the LH pulses. Some rare hypothalamic syndromes, such as Prader–Willi syndrome, are associated with both obesity and hypogonadotrophic hypogonadism. Another possible mechanism to explain the aetiology of low testosterone levels and the subsequent insulin resistance in obese men is hyperoestrogenaemia. There are increased serum levels of oestradiol and oestrone in obese men, which is primarily as a result of increased peripheral conversion of androgens to oestrogens through the action of the enzyme aromatase in the adipose tissue. This increase in serum oestrogen concentration is, however, not accompanied by overt signs of feminization. It is therefore possible that the increased oestradiol levels contribute to the insulin resistance in obese men.

Some chest diseases are associated with infertility (e.g. congenital absence of the vas deferens may be associated with cystic fibrosis or Kartagener syndrome with dextrocardia) and might be elicited at the time of the examination.

Men with severe androgen deficiency of prepubertal origin will have a high-pitched voice, small soft testes and small penis, lack of pubic and axillary hair, and decreased muscle mass. They are often tall, with a large arm span that exceeds their height. If hypogonadism develops after puberty, the skin becomes fine and body and facial hair diminish. There may be gynaecomastia, as in Klinefelter's syndrome, although the phenotype in Klinefelter's syndrome can vary quite widely. Gynaecomastia may also occur with hyperthyroidism, liver disease, oestrogen- or human chorionic gonadotrophin (hCG)-producing tumours and as a side-effect of some drugs, such as cimetidine, spironolactone and digoxin. Abdominal examination should reveal the presence of abnormal masses, hernias or scars from herniorrhaphy. Genital examination is best performed in a warm room with the patient standing. This examination only needs to be performed if there are sexual difficulties, symptoms or signs of hypogonadism, or abnormalities with the semen analysis. A full neurological examination is also required when there are problems with sexual function.

Investigations

Attendance at the fertility clinic should be utilized for general health screening and preconception counselling. Particular attention should be paid to body weight, blood pressure, urinalysis, cervical cytology and rubella immunity.

Ovarian function

Regular menstrual cycles are a sign of ovulation in 95% of the cycles. However, the regularity of the cycles alone is not enough to characterize ovarian function. The number of follicles in the ovaries decreases from birth, resulting in a slow decline in fertility from the age of 30 onwards. This decline parallels the reduction in the number and quality of the follicles and oocytes. The first sign of reduced ovarian activity is the shortening of the follicular phase, which reduces the length of the ovulatory cycle. The decrease in the number of follicles is followed by hormonal changes: inhibin B is produced by the small antral follicles, and as their numbers decline, the ovarian output of inhibin B decreases. This is paralleled by a rise in follicle-stimulating hormone (FSH) level.

Tests of ovarian reserve include measurement of the early follicular phase FSH (normal <10 IU/L) and oestradiol levels (days 1–3 of cycle; normal <75 pmol/L) to determine the FSH:oestradiol ratio, measurement of day 3 inhibin B (normal >45 pg/mL) or antimüllerian hormone levels (normal >15.7 pmol/L), and undertaking early follicular phase antral follicle count. Other options include dynamic tests to evaluate the ovaries during clomiphene citrate challenge or gonadotrophin stimulation. These tests will help to determine the most suitable treatment and are useful in counselling the couple.

An elevated FSH level indicates reduced ovarian reserve. In general terms, if FSH levels are greater than 10 IU/L the ovaries are unlikely to be ovulating regularly and will also be resistant to exogenous stimulation. Levels greater than 25 IU/L are suggestive of the menopause or premature ovarian failure. An elevated serum concentration of LH may suggest that the patient has PCOS. Other causes of an elevated LH are the mid-cycle surge and ovarian failure. The association of amenorrhoea with very low levels of FSH and LH (usually <2 IU/L) suggests pituitary failure or hypogonadotrophic hypogonadism. Gonadotrophin measurements are best interpreted together with the findings of a pelvic ultrasound scan, as these will provide the diagnosis in most cases.

Ovulation can be documented in several ways. The easiest is to measure a mid-luteal phase progesterone level. The clinical menstrual history will give fairly reliable information about the presence or absence of ovulation. A progesterone concentration greater than 30 nmol/L suggests ovulation. If the progesterone is 15–30 nmol/L, then ovulation may be occurring but the timing of the measurement may have been incorrect. It is then necessary to check the timing of the blood test to subsequent menstruation (the test should be performed 7 days prior to menstruation) and repeated in the following cycle, sometimes with serial measurements.

Basal body temperature (BBT) charts work on the rationale that progesterone will raise BBT by 0.2–0.5°C, although between 10 and 75% of ovulatory cycles fail to show such a degree of rise in BBT. BBT charts are therefore a source of considerable stress and do not provide a prospective indication of the day of ovulation. Commercially available kits that detect the presence of LH in the urine are expensive and may also cause unnecessary anxiety but are more accurate in detecting the LH surge and timing of ovulation.

When the cycles are irregular, other hormonal measurements such as testosterone, dehydroepiandrosterone sulphate (DHEAS), 17-hydroxyprogesterone, cortisol, prolactin and thyroid function tests may be necessary. If the results of any of these tests are considered abnormal, appropriate biochemical and imaging studies should be conducted.

Tubal assessment

When ovarian function and semen analysis are normal, tubal status should be investigated, particularly in women with a history of pelvic surgery, sexually transmitted infections or tubo-ovarian disease. Laparoscopy is the gold standard for the evaluation of tubal patency, during which peritubal adhesions, the ovaries, the peritoneum and the liver surface should be assessed and endometriosis (Fig. 7.3) excluded.

Other procedures, such as hysterosalpingography or hysterosalpingo contrast sonography, can also be used to assess tubal patency. They are useful in evaluating isthmic (proximal) and total fimbrial (distal) blockage, but are less helpful than laparoscopy in the diagnosis of partial tubal obstruction, peritubal adhesions or other contributory factors of tubal infertility such as severe endometriosis and pelvic adhesions, from either non-tubal intra-abdominal infection or previous surgery.[8]

Uterine evaluation

Transvaginal ultrasound is a routine part of the infertility work-up and is used to assess uterine outline, position and morphology, and the adnexa. Fibroids, polyps, congenital anomalies, abnormalities of the endometrium, hydrosalpinx and ovarian masses can be detected. It is also possible to instil a small volume of normal saline into the uterine cavity using a small catheter to more accurately delineate its outline and the precise size

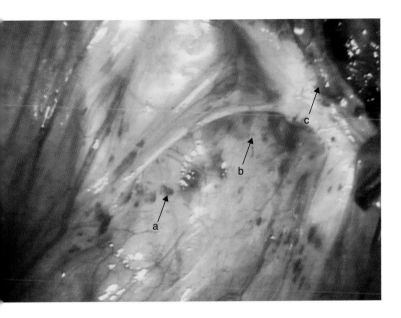

Figure 7.3
Laparoscopic view of the pelvis, with different manifestations of endometriosis. **(a)** Haemorrhagic lesions with increased peritoneal vascularity. **(b)** Peritoneal pouch (pocket) near right uterosacral ligament. **(c)** Haemorrhagic vesicles, right uterosacral ligament.

and location of any intracavity focal lesions. Additional information may be obtained during hysteroscopy with direct visualization of the uterine cavity. Three-dimensional ultrasound has in recent years become a valuable medical imaging modality. Recent advances in three-dimensional ultrasound have made accurate non-invasive assessment of pelvic organs possible, with potential improvements in the assessment and management of infertility problems. A number of uterine abnormalities have been linked to infertility and/or spontaneous abortion, such as congenital uterine structural anomalies, fibroids, polyps and synechiae. Although each of these conditions may contribute to infertility, they are also seen in association with pregnancy; a causal link has therefore not been established.

Chlamydia *testing*

Testing for *chlamydia* may be undertaken with swabs or serology. *Chlamydia* serology is the best initial screen for tubal disease. A raised titre (>1:256) correctly predicts tubal damage in 90% of cases, over half of which give no history of PID.[9] High antibody titres may indicate current or previous tubal infection. Treatment does not correct tubal damage but prevents reactivation if uterine instrumentation is performed.

Chlamydia screening may help identify women whose tubal status should be tested early in the investigative process and by a laparoscopy rather than the other methods. If the screen test is positive, the woman and her partner should be referred for suitable treatment and contact tracing. Swabbing for *Chlamydia* identifies active disease and when positive is an indication for treatment of the sexual partners and contact tracing.

Postcoital test

The postcoital test was introduced to provide information about the interaction between sperm and cervical mucus.[10] However, review of the literature does not support its use in today's practice.

Semen analysis

The evaluation of the male partner starts with a semen analysis, which should be performed after 3 days of abstinence. The volume of the semen, sperm number, motility and morphology assessment complete the examination. The World Health Organization (WHO) criteria for a normal semen analysis are outlined in Table 7.3.[11] When one or several of these parameters are abnormal, the analysis should be repeated in 3 months, and further tests may be necessary. Azoospermia (absence of sperm) represents a barrier to natural conception, and further tests are necessary to determine the exact cause and prognosis. Clinicians must be cautious in interpreting low sperm values, especially if they are only mildly reduced below the range considered normal, as there are no data on where we should draw thresholds for normal and abnormal sperm parameters. Nineteen per cent of men in an infertile population will have a sperm count less than 20 million/mL, but so will 8% of men in a fertile population.[12]

Trial sperm wash

The increasing number of men showing poor semen quality prompted the development of the trial sperm wash. This assessment is usually performed when the sperm concentration is 10 million/mL or less to help in deciding which treatment options are most suitable for the couple. The aim of the sperm preparation is to select motile and functionally competent spermatozoa from the ejaculate to improve the fertilization potential of the sample.

Table 7.3: Normal semen parameters

Parameter	Value
Volume	2.0 mL
pH	7.2–8.0
Sperm concentration	20×10^6/mL
Total sperm count	40×10^6 per ejaculate
Motility (within 60 min of ejaculation)	25% with rapid progression (A)
	50% with forward progression (A and B)
Vitality	75% live (A, B and C)
	25% dead (D)
Morphology	30% normal forms
White blood cells	$<1 \times 10^6$/mL
Sperm antibodies	<50%

(From World Health Organization 1999,[11] with permission.)

Endocrine investigations in men

Gonadal status (testosterone, LH, FSH), prolactin and thyroid function should be measured in men with oligospermia (count less than 10 million sperm/mL) or if there are signs or symptoms suggestive of either androgen deficiency or endocrine disease. Serum testosterone levels undergo diurnal variation, with the highest levels in the morning. The normal range is 10–35 nmol/L. Recommendations for the evaluation of hyperprolactinaemia and male gonadal disease are given in Chapters 1 and 6, respectively. Normal serum concentrations of FSH and LH are less than 10 IU/L. The combination of azoospermia with normal levels of testosterone, FSH and LH indicates a mechanical obstruction and warrants urological assessment. An elevated FSH level indicates germinal cell insufficiency or, if combined with an elevated LH concentration and a low testosterone level, primary testicular failure. Low serum concentrations of all three hormones indicate hypothalamic or pituitary insufficiency, which may be amenable to hormonal therapy with hCG and FSH. Serum prolactin and thyroid function should be measured when testosterone and gonadotrophin levels are low or when there is gynaecomastia or there are signs of thyroid disease.

Men with primary gonadal failure or with severe male factor infertility (sperm count less than 5 million/mL) should undergo genetic testing (karyotype, Y chromosome microdeletions, cystic fibrosis gene mutation analysis). The incidence of sex chromosome or Y chromosome abnormalities is about 15% among men with azoospermia.

TREATMENT OF THE INFERTILE COUPLE

Tubal and uterine disease

The role of microsurgery for proximal tubal obstruction is debatable, as no randomized controlled trials or controlled observational studies are available to compare microsurgery with no treatment or with in vitro fertilization (IVF). Surgery for pelvic and tubal disease and its outcome depends on the age of the woman, the duration of and factors associated with infertility, and the availability of appropriate equipment and skilled surgeons, and is also linked closely to the severity of the damage, with better results achieved in those with filmy adhesions and limited damage. Most pregnancies occur between 12 and 14 months after surgery, and if no conception has occurred IVF would be indicated. Pregnancy rates after tubal surgery are comparable with those resulting from IVF, while the incidence of ectopic pregnancy varies from 8 to 23% following surgery for proximal and distal occlusion, respectively. The choice between surgery and IVF as the primary treatment will depend on careful patient selection according to the individual's clinical circumstances and involving the couple in the decision-making process.

Tubal catheterization or cannulation for proximal tubal blockage may be achieved using either a radiographic approach (selective salpingography combined with tubal cannulation) or hysteroscopically. The National Institute for Health and Clinical

Excellence (NICE) has recommended that in women with proximal obstruction these techniques may be alternative treatment options, as they improve the chance of pregnancy.

Women with fibroids have lower spontaneous pregnancy rates than those without them or with other causes of infertility. Myomectomy appears to improve the pregnancy rate, although its impact on live birth rate is uncertain. Women with fibroids may also have a reduced pregnancy rate following assisted reproduction treatment (ART). The role of uterine artery embolization in improving the reproductive outcome of women with fibroids remains to be determined. Women with uterine septa and adhesions may benefit from surgery by improving the live term birth rate and reducing the miscarriage rate following spontaneous or ART conception.

Patients with endometriosis: medical and surgical treatment

Medical treatment of minimal and mild endometriosis with ovulation suppression agents (medroxyprogesterone, gestrinone, combined oral contraceptives, gonadotrophin-releasing hormone, GnRH, analogues) does not improve clinical pregnancy rates in women with endometriosis-associated infertility and should not be offered.

Women with minimal or mild endometriosis benefit from laparoscopic ablation or resection of endometriotic deposits plus adhesiolysis, and their ongoing pregnancy and live birth rates increase compared with diagnostic laparoscopy only. In women who have mild endometriosis as their only infertility factor, the pregnancy rate is higher after laser laparoscopy and laparotomy compared with medical treatment. However, the benefits of surgery should be balanced against the risks of general anaesthesia and surgical complications.

In women with moderate or severe endometriosis, laparoscopic surgery may improve the spontaneous pregnancy rate compared with laparotomy. In women with ovarian endometriotic cysts, NICE has recommended that these women should be offered laparoscopic cystectomy as opposed to drainage and coagulation, as it improves their spontaneous pregnancy rate. However, the value of surgery in women selected for IVF or intracytoplasmic sperm injection (ICSI) cycles is debated and is not supported by the available evidence. Postoperative medical treatment does not improve pregnancy rates and is not recommended.

Management of ovulatory dysfunction

Women with WHO group 1 ovulation disorders (hypothalamic–pituitary failure, amenorrhoea or hypogonadotrophic hypogonadism) should be offered pulsatile GnRH or gonadotrophins with LH, because these are effective in inducing ovulation.

Women with a BMI of more than 29 kg/m^2 are likely to take longer to conceive, and those who are not ovulating should be informed that losing weight would recommence ovulation and is likely to increase their chance of conception. Equally, women who have a BMI of less than 19 kg/m^2 and who have irregular or absent menstruation should be advised that increasing body weight is likely to improve their chance of conception.

Ovulation induction aims to achieve unifollicular ovulation in the correction of anovulatory infertility, the commonest cause of which is PCOS. In these women, NICE guidelines advise the use of antioestrogens (clomiphene citrate or tamoxifen) for up to 12 months as a first-line therapy, because it is likely to induce ovulation. The cumulative pregnancy rates continue to rise after six treatment cycles before reaching a plateau, and are comparable with those of the normal fertile population. It has been suggested that at least one cycle of therapy should be monitored with ultrasound to ensure that response is assessed and that drug doses are adjusted to minimize the risk of multiple pregnancy. Adverse effects of antioestrogens include hot flushes, ovarian hyperstimulation syndrome (OHSS), abdominal discomfort and multiple pregnancies. Women who ovulate with clomiphene citrate but who do not conceive should be offered clomiphene citrate-stimulated intrauterine insemination (IUI).

A Cochrane Database systematic review of 15 randomized controlled trials concluded that in women with clomiphene-resistant PCOS and a mean BMI above 25 kg/m^2, metformin as a single agent was not found to increase clinical pregnancy rate when compared with placebo.[13] However, treatment with both metformin and clomiphene citrate did increase clinical pregnancy rate compared with clomiphene citrate alone, hence these women should be offered the combined treatment. Metformin as a single agent was found to induce ovulation when compared with placebo, and in combination with clomiphene citrate was also effective in inducing ovulation compared with clomiphene citrate alone. The effectiveness of pulsatile GnRH in women with clomiphene citrate-resistant PCOS is uncertain and is therefore not recommended outside a research context.

Women prescribed metformin should be informed of the side-effects associated with its use, such as nausea, vomiting and other gastrointestinal disturbances. To minimize these, patients should initially be commenced on a low dose (500 mg once daily), building up gradually to a maintenance dose of 500 mg twice daily and subsequently, if tolerated, a maximally effective dose of 1 g twice daily. If these women remain non-responsive, they may be offered laparoscopic ovarian drilling, because it is as effective as gonadotrophin treatment and is not associated with an increased risk of multiple pregnancies. However, this treatment is associated with surgical risks, its benefits wane with time and the long-term effects are poorly understood.

Treatment with gonadotrophins, human menopausal gonadotrophin, urinary FSH and recombinant FSH are equally effective in achieving pregnancy, and consideration should be given to minimizing cost when prescribing. The use of adjuvant growth hormone treatment with GnRH agonist and/or human menopausal gonadotrophin during ovulation induction in women with PCOS who do not respond to clomiphene citrate is not recommended, as it does not improve pregnancy rates. Women who are offered ovulation induction with gonadotrophins should be informed about the risk of multiple pregnancy and OHSS before starting treatment. Women with ovulatory disorders due to hyperprolactinaemia should be offered treatment with dopamine agonists such as bromocriptine or cabergoline (see Chapter 1).

Ovarian ultrasound monitoring to measure follicular size and number should be an integral part of patient management during gonadotrophin therapy to reduce the risk of multiple pregnancy and OHSS. Women who are offered ovulation induction should be informed that a possible association between ovulation induction therapy and ovarian cancer remains uncertain.

The role of intrauterine insemination: homologous and donor sperm

Intrauterine insemination involves timed insemination of sperm into the uterus in natural (unstimulated) cycles or following stimulation of the ovaries using oral antioestrogens or gonadotrophins. It is often undertaken following unsuccessful ovulation induction treatment in women with patent tubes but who suffer from unexplained infertility, ovulatory dysfunction or endometriosis, or when there is a degree of sperm factor dysfunction (count and motility) that requires sperm preparation prior to insemination. Success rate following IUI is dependent on:

- the age of the woman
- the number of developing follicles
- the endometrial thickness
- the duration and type of infertility
- the progressive motility of the sperm sample.

While there is debate over the true relevance of some of these factors, it is clear that the number of developing follicles is important, with a multifollicular response improving pregnancy rates. This multifollicular response is only possible if controlled ovarian stimulation is performed.

In male factor infertility, there are no set criteria for minimal sperm parameters to be used for insemination; however, it is recognized that a sperm preparation of $>2 \times 10^6$ motile sperm per mL is sufficient for IUI. When male factor is the sole cause of infertility, the pregnancy rate is similar following IUI in natural and stimulated cycles, but on both occasions better than timed intercourse. However, when multiple factors are present, stimulated IUI improves the pregnancy rate (although multiple pregnancy rates increase). Multiple pregnancies contribute significantly to perinatal mortality, morbidity and National Health Service costs.

In women with unexplained infertility, controlled ovarian stimulation and IUI results in higher pregnancy rates compared with natural cycles or with intracervical insemination only. Similarly, gonadotrophin-stimulated IUI increases the chance of pregnancy compared with gonadotrophins plus timed intercourse. In women with minimal or mild endometriosis, pregnancy and live birth rates are significantly higher with stimulated IUI cycles, although this is again associated with high multiple pregnancy rate. It is hypothesized that oocyte quality or other factors associated with endometriosis adversely affect the spontaneous pregnancy rate.

IVF and ICSI treatments

The decision to offer IVF or ICSI treatment should be based on the results of previous investigations and the precise diagnosis and duration of infertility, taking into consideration the probability of spontaneous pregnancy without treatment. However, a number of studies have shown higher pregnancy and live birth rates when couples resort to IVF treatment sooner rather than later. Current indications for IVF and ICSI treatments are summarized in Box 7.4.

Procedures involved in IVF and ICSI

In vitro fertilization treatment involves a number of principal steps that have remained relatively unchanged over the past 25 years. These include:

- superovulation (commonly called ovulation induction)
- oocyte retrieval
- IVF
- embryo transfer
- luteal phase support.

However, considerable refinements have taken place over the past decades, leading to significantly improved pregnancy rates.

Controlled ovarian stimulation

Superovulation protocols have evolved over the years – from the use of clomiphene citrate with or without gonadotrophins in the early years to more complex regimens using GnRH agonist and antagonists with subcutaneously administered recombinant gonadotrophins. Typical regimens now comprise a long down-regulation protocol using GnRH agonist with subsequent recombinant FSH or human menopausal gonadotrophin injections to induce scheduled follicular recruitment and growth of a cohort of mature follicles. Recently introduced GnRH antagonists have some advantages over the agonist group, namely shorter duration of treatment, absence of a flare-up effect and of pituitary down-regulation when used for a short interval, and lower risk of OHSS. However, they have been associated with lower clinical pregnancy rates. Follicular development must be monitored closely using ultrasound scans with or without hormone assays.

Box 7.4: Indications for in vitro fertilization or intracytoplasmic sperm injection treatments

- Tubal disease when surgery has not been successful or has been considered inappropriate
- Male factor infertility that is not correctable through other measures
- Endometriosis when other treatments have been deemed unsuitable or been unsuccessful
- Unexplained infertility when less invasive measures such as medical treatment or intrauterine insemination have not been successful
- Ovulatory disorders when other options have been exhausted and unsuccessful
- Egg donation due to premature ovarian failure or poor oocyte quality
- Intracytoplasmic sperm injection is indicated when there is severe impairment of sperm quality or number, or obstructive or non-obstructive azoospermia, and when previous in vitro fertilization treatment was accompanied by failed or very poor fertilization

Oocyte retrieval

Luteinizing hormone is given 34–37 h before oocyte retrieval to trigger the final stages of oocyte maturation. The transvaginal route is now the accepted standard technique for oocyte retrievals (Fig. 7.4), and the procedure is carried out mostly under conscious sedation for pain relief, administered by trained staff in the unit without the need for an anaesthetist as long as they follow guidelines published by the Academy of Medical Royal Colleges. NICE guidelines recommend that women undergoing transvaginal retrieval should be offered conscious sedation, as it is a safe and effective method.

Embryo transfer: day of transfer and technique

Embryo transfers may be carried out on day 2 or 3, or day 4 or 5, after oocyte retrieval. Ultrasound-guided embryo transfer has been shown in meta-analyses to increase the clinical pregnancy rates when compared with clinical touch technique, with the patient resting for about 20 min afterwards before resuming normal activity.

Luteal phase support

Superovulation protocols including GnRH agonists or antagonists would benefit from hCG and intramuscular progesterone supplementation, which result in higher clinical pregnancy and live birth rates. However, hCG is associated with a higher risk of OHSS and is generally not routinely recommended.

Success rates: IVF and ICSI

In 2006, the Human Fertilization and Embryology Authority (HFEA) reported the outcomes of 29 688 patients undergoing 38 264 IVF cycles between 1 April 2003 and 31 March 2004 and resulting in the successful births of 10 242 children. The average live birth rates for IVF treatment using fresh eggs ranged from 28.2% for women under the age of 35 years to 10.6% for those aged 40–42 years. The live birth rates following frozen embryo replacement cycles ranged from 16.8 to 6.9% for the same age groups,

Figure 7.4
Transvaginal oocyte collection showing needle within a follicle: **(a)** follicles, **(b)** needle tip, **(c)** ovarian tissue.

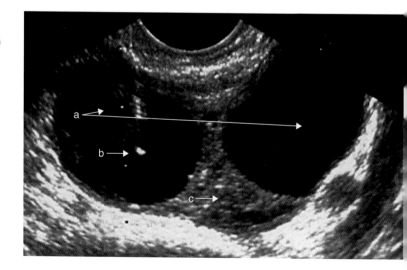

respectively. The multiple birth rate (twins and triplets) following fresh and frozen cycles for the same period was 23.6%.

Ectopic pregnancy rates based on analysis of 110 538 IVF treatment cycles that were registered by the HFEA between January 1995 and March 1999 and involved use of the woman's own eggs and fresh embryo transfer showed an overall ectopic pregnancy rate per treatment cycle of 0.5% (18–25 years, 0.9%; >35 years, less than 0.3%).

Miscarriage rates based on analysis of the above 110 538 IVF treatment cycles showed an overall miscarriage rate per treatment cycle of 2.7%, while the miscarriage rate in women aged more than 35 years was 2.4%. Calculations based on numbers of pregnancies indicate a miscarriage rate per pregnancy of:

- 10.5% at 30 years
- 13.1% at 35 years
- 22.7% at 40 years
- 40.7% at 43 years.

These rates are comparable with those following spontaneous pregnancies.

Clinical factors affecting success

Analysis of the HFEA database and other national surveys has demonstrated that outcomes are affected by the following factors.

- Increasing duration of infertility significantly decreases live birth rate, irrespective of age.
- Male or multiple infertility factors are associated with lowest outcomes, but those with tubal, endocrine and unexplained infertility have comparable success rate with the probability of natural conception in young, fertile couples. Women with hydrosalpinges will benefit from pre-IVF salpingectomy and, equally, those with secondary infertility have higher pregnancy and live birth rates than those with primary infertility.
- Pregnancy and live birth rates following IVF decrease with advancing female age, irrespective of whether fresh or frozen embryos are used, with optimal treatment age between 23 and 38 years. Lowest pregnancy rates occur in women aged 40 or above. However, older women with good ovarian response, producing more than three embryos suitable for transfer, may have a pregnancy rate similar to that of younger patients, whereas cycles yielding less than three embryos have a poor prognosis.
- The transfer of a higher number of embryos results in a higher number of fetuses that might be born. This higher multiple pregnancy risk has its health risks on mother and babies, as well as economic implications. At present, the HFEA guidance is that no more than two embryos should be transferred during any one cycle of IVF. There are indications that an elective single embryo transfer policy should be adopted to further lower the risk of multiple pregnancy.
- Each IVF attempt has a similar success rate to the other; however, with increased number of treatment cycles advancing female age determines the outcome, and hence lower pregnancy and live birth rates may be observed.

- There is no evidence to suggest that tubal embryo transfer, zygote intrafallopian transfer or gamete intrafallopian transfer result in higher pregnancy or live birth rates.
- There are also differences in the success rates between the various centres.

Lifestyle factors

- Alcohol consumption in excess of one unit per day reduces the effectiveness of ART.
- Smoking by either partner has a negative effect on the outcome of treatment.
- Caffeine consumption has an adverse effect on outcome.
- NICE has recommended that the BMI of the female partner should be 19–30 kg/m^2 before commencing fertility treatment, as the likelihood of success is reduced outside this range.

Oocyte donation

Egg donation is an effective treatment for women with primary or secondary premature ovarian failure, gonadal dysgenesis such as Turner's syndrome, following oophorectomy, and chemo- or radiotherapy-related ovarian failure, and when repeated failure of fertilization is attributed to poor oocyte quality. In addition, oocyte donation might be employed in women with markedly diminished ovarian reserve or to avoid the risk of transmission of a genetic disorder in cases in which the carrier status of both partners is known.

High pregnancy rates have been reported following oocyte donation for Turner's syndrome patients. However, these women have a significantly higher biochemical pregnancy rate and early miscarriages, and lower clinical pregnancy and delivery rates, when compared with other women with premature ovarian failure. An important factor in the establishment of pregnancy is an endometrial thickness of greater than 6.5 mm. Other factors include the number of previous natural conceptions and live births, and the fertilization rate, but not advancing female age. Women with Turner's syndrome should also be screened before their treatment to exclude phenotypic manifestations of the syndrome that might jeopardize successful pregnancy, including aortic dilation and cardiac lesions. All oocyte donors should be screened for both infectious and genetic diseases in accordance with guidance issued by the HFEA, and in view of the considerable emotional and social effects on both the donor and the recipient, counselling must be offered for all involved by someone who is independent of the treatment unit.

Male factor infertility

Gonadotrophins have been shown to improve fertility in men with hypogonadotrophic hypogonadism (e.g. secondary testicular failure, Kallmann's syndrome). Pulsatile GnRH may be as effective in enhancing sperm production in some of these men. Injections of hCG are administered thrice weekly, with regular monitoring of testosterone response. FSH is added thereafter to induce spermatogenesis. The response is variable and depends on the precise cause, severity, time of onset and clinical features, and it may take months or years for sperm counts to increase to within the normal range.

However, no other drugs have been shown to be effective for idiopathic sperm abnormalities or antisperm antibodies. Furthermore, antibiotic therapy should not be used routinely for leucospermia unless a specific pathogen is isolated. Surgery for obstructive azoospermia improves fertility and is an appropriate alternative to percutaneous epididymal sperm aspiration (PESA) and IVF. However, surgery for varicoceles does not improve pregnancy rates. In men with anejaculation or retroejaculation, penile electrovibration or transrectal electroejaculation helps to retrieve motile sperm for IUI, IVF or ICSI, depending on its quality, and is preferred by many to medical therapy with its substantial side-effects. Should either or both approaches fail, PESA and IVF remain an appropriate alternative for these men. Anxiolytic drugs and/or sildenafil are recommended when ejaculatory failure is associated with erectile dysfunction of psychogenic origin.

Risks associated with assisted reproduction treatment

At each stage of ART, complications may occur, and some may even be life-threatening. Psychological and emotional effects are present before, during and after treatment and can adversely affect the couple's relationship. They include concerns on the outcome of treatment, effects on the baby, multiple pregnancy and the risk of cancer.

The incidence of treatment-related complications varies. Adverse events during oocyte recovery and OHSS occur in 1.3–8.3% of cases. Operative complications associated with transvaginal oocyte retrieval include haemorrhage at the puncture site, serious intra-abdominal bleeding, bowel and ureteric injury, and pelvic infection. However, the most serious complication associated with ART is OHSS. Moderate or severe OHSS occurs in 0.5–10% of stimulation cycles, and up to 1% of all patients require hospitalization. Identification of risk factors before treatment (young age, PCOS or thin body stature) and during treatment (excessive follicular development on scan and high oestrogen levels) is critical to the prediction and prevention of this life-threatening complication. Several strategies have been employed to prevent the development of OHSS, including use of a low starting gonadotrophin dose or dose reduction during treatment, close monitoring, coasting (withholding gonadotrophins for 24–64 h before the hCG injection), elective cryopreservation of all embryos, intravenous albumin administration during oocyte retrieval and avoidance of hCG for luteal phase support.

Treatment of established moderate or severe OHSS requires close monitoring of symptoms, biochemical profile and fluid balance. This may necessitate admission to hospital and treatment in a high-dependency unit if necessary. Additional measures for pain relief, thromboprophylaxis and paracentesis may be required.

Concerns have been expressed on the risk of ovarian, breast and endometrial cancers in women undergoing ovulation induction or IVF treatment. At present, there is no evidence of an increased risk of breast and ovarian cancer in women who have undergone IVF as compared with subfertile women. There does seem to be a small increased risk of endometrial cancer in those exposed to IVF, but this is also apparent in the unexposed group, suggesting a subfertility-related effect.

Obstetric complications are a further hazard of ART and extend throughout pregnancy itself and on to the peri- and neonatal periods. An overall early pregnancy loss of around 20% is comparable with spontaneous pregnancies, but there is a slightly increased ectopic pregnancy rate. A meta-analysis of 15 singleton pregnancy studies encompassing 1.9 million spontaneous and over 12 000 IVF pregnancies showed significantly increased rates of perinatal mortality, preterm delivery, low birth weight, placenta praevia, gestational diabetes and pre-eclampsia for IVF pregnancies. High multiple pregnancy rate following IVF is a significant contributor to adverse obstetric and perinatal outcomes, hence the HFEA guidance on reducing the number of embryos transferred to two only.

Acknowledgement

The publication of the National Collaborating Centre for Women's and Children's Health clinical guideline on the assessment and treatment of fertility problems on behalf of NICE has considerably influenced UK practice. The authors of this chapter have attempted to remain within the parameters of this guideline, which inevitably formed a principal source of the manuscript, and where appropriate presented alternative views based on more recent evidence.

References

1. Hull MGR, Cahill DJ 1998 Female infertility. Endocrinol Metab Clin North Am 27(4): 851–876
2. Trussell J, Wilson C 1985 Sterility in a population with natural fertility. Popul Stud 29: 269–286
3. Cahill D, Wardle PJ 2002 Management of infertility. Br Med J 325: 28–32
4. Wang JX, Davies M, Norman RJ 2000 Body mass and probability of pregnancy during assisted reproduction treatment: retrospective study. Br Med J 321: 1320–1321
5. Van der Spuy ZM, Steer PJ, McCusker M et al. 1988 Outcome of pregnancy in underweight women after spontaneous and induced ovulation. Br Med J 296: 962–965
6. Hamilton-Fairley D, Kiddy D, Watson H et al. 1992 Association of moderate obesity with poor pregnancy outcome in women with polycystic ovary syndrome treated with low dose gonadotrophins. Br J Obstet Gynaecol 99: 128–131
7. Clark AM, Thornley B, Thomlinson L et al. 1998 Weight loss in obese infertile women results in improvement in reproductive outcome for all forms of fertility treatment. Hum Reprod 13: 1502–1505
8. Chen YM, Ott DJ, Pittaway DE et al. 1988 Efficacy of hysterosalpingography in evaluating tubal and peritubal disease in 200 patients with infertility. Rays 13: 27–32
9. Akande VA, Hunt LP, Cahill DJ et al. 2003 Tubal damage in infertile women: prediction using *Chlamydia* serology. Hum Reprod 18(9): 1841–1847
10. Overstreet JW 1986 Evaluation of sperm–cervical mucus interaction. Fertil Steril 45: 324–326
11. World Health Organization 1999 WHO laboratory manual for the examination of human semen and sperm–cervical mucus interaction, 4th edn. Cambridge University Press, Cambridge
12. MacLeod J, Gold RZ 1951 The male factor in fertility and infertility. II. Spermatozoon counts in 1000 men of known fertility and in 1000 cases of infertile marriage. J Urol 66: 436–449
13. Lord JM, Flight IH, Norman RJ 2003 Insulin-sensitising drugs (metformin, troglitazone, rosiglitazone, pioglitazone, D-chiro-inositol) for polycystic ovary syndrome. Cochrane Database Syst Rev 3: CD003053

Further reading

Academy of Medical Royal Colleges 2001 Implementing and ensuring safe practice for health procedures in adults. Report of an intercollegiate working party chaired by the Royal College of Anaesthetists. AORMC, London

Amso NN, Shaw RW 2003 Assisted reproduction treatments. In: Shaw RW, Soutter WP, Stanton SL (eds) Gynaecology, 3rd edn. Churchill Livingstone, London, pp. 317–342

Cheong YC, Li TC 2005 Evidence-based management of tubal disease and infertility. Curr Obstet Gynecol 15: 306–313

Heijnen EMEW, Eijkemans MJC, Hughes EG et al. 2006 A meta-analysis of outcomes of conventional IVF in women with PCOS. Hum Reprod Update 12: 13–21

Mathur R, Evbuomwan I, Jenkins J 2005 Prevention and management of ovarian hyperstimulation syndrome. Curr Obstet Gynaecol 15: 132–138

National Collaborating Centre for Women's and Children's Health 2004 Fertility assessment and treatment for people with fertility problems. RCOG Press, London

Ola B, Ledger WE 2005 In vitro fertilisation. IVF treatments. Curr Obstet Gynecol 15: 314–323

Seif MW 2005 Managing disorders of ovulation: a model for evidence-based practice. Curr Opin Obstet Gynecol 17: 403–404

Somigliana E, Vercillini P, Vigano P et al. 2006 Should endometrioma be treated before IVF–ICSI cycles. Hum Reprod Update 12: 306–313

SELF-ASSESSMENT

Patient 1

A 32-year-old woman with a history of oligomenorrhoea, hirsutism and weight gain is referred to you, having failed to spontaneously conceive for over 2 years.

Question

1. What factors would you wish to elicit in the history? What features should you look for during your examination? Which biochemical and radiological tests should you request?

Answer

1. Duration of symptoms. Other associated features (e.g. galactorrhoea, visual disturbance, headaches). Any features of virilization from history (e.g. deepening of the voice) or examination (e.g. increased muscle bulk, clitoromegaly)? Has the patient been hypertensive or diabetic? Does she have symptoms of easy bruising or proximal myopathy? Is there a relevant family history? Is she a smoker? Has there been any previous obstetric or gynaecological history of note, such as previous sexually transmitted disease or PID? Look for features of Cushing's syndrome and hypothyroidism on examination. Check visual fields and examine for galactorrhoea.

Check prolactin, thyroid function tests, and gonadotrophin and androgen measurement (testosterone, DHEAS, androstenedione). Consider tests for Cushing's syndrome (urinary free cortisol, dexamethasone suppression testing, salivary cortisol) and late-onset congenital adrenal hyperplasia (early morning follicular phase 17-hydroxyprogesterone). Perform urinalysis and measure fasting glucose. Request ovarian ultrasound scan if PCOS is suspected. Request magnetic resonance imaging (MRI) of pituitary gland if prolactin level is persistently elevated. Consider ovarian/adrenal MRI scans if testosterone is greater than 5 nmol/L.

The patient has a long history of oligomenorrhoea, dating back to the menarche. There is no galactorrhoea, visual disturbance or headache. Her hirsutism is mainly confined to the face and umbilicus, and there are no signs of virilization, Cushing's syndrome or hypothyroidism. Her serum prolactin, thyroid function tests and 17-hydroxyprogesterone are normal and testosterone is 2.8 nmol/L, with a modestly raised androstenedione (14 nmol/L; normal range 4–10 nmol/L). Screening for Cushing's syndrome is negative. Ovarian ultrasonography demonstrates 12 follicles of less than 10 mm in diameter at the periphery, with increased central stromal echogenicity. The patient's BMI is 34 kg/m².

Question

2. What is the likely diagnosis? What would be your initial management strategy? How would you counsel her?

Answer

2. Polycystic ovary syndrome. Recommend weight loss and exercise, as well as smoking cessation if the patient is a smoker. Check rubella immunity. Begin folic acid (400 µg daily). Check for male factor infertility. Commence clomiphene citrate in the first instance if lifestyle measures are ineffective. If the patient fails to ovulate with clomiphene, then can add metformin. Counsel her that fertility is reduced and that weight loss is essential for improving fertility and other features of PCOS. Additionally, fertility can be improved with strategies comprising insulin sensitization, ovulation induction and/or IVF.

Despite clomiphene and metformin therapy, the patient does not become pregnant after 12 months.

Question

3. What other therapeutic options are there?

Answer

3. Gonadotrophin therapy with or without IUI, laparoscopic ovarian diathermy and IVF.

Patient 2

A 34-year-old woman and her 35-year-old partner are being seen in the fertility clinic with a 4-year history of primary infertility.

Question

1. What relevant information in the couple's history would you require, and what examination would you need to undertake in the initial assessment?

Answer

1. The female history would involve an assessment of previous contraception use and any associated problems (such as lost coil), previous pregnancies and outcome, medical history (e.g. pelvic infection, Crohn disease), surgical history (e.g. ovarian cyst, appendectomy), gynaecological history (cone biopsy, cervical smear history), current medical illness, drug history (prescribed and misuse), diet, smoking and alcohol consumption, galactorrhoea, hirsutism, menstrual regularity and menorrhagia, dysmenorrhoea, intermenstrual or postcoital bleeding, preovulatory cervical mucus recognition, and coital frequency and timing.

Examination would be general, with BMI, signs of endocrine disease, and abdominal examination. An ultrasound scan of the pelvis should be performed to assess uterine and ovarian morphology and to exclude any adnexal lesions such as hydrosalpinges.

The male history would assess occupation (exposure to excessive heat or toxins), medical history such as mumps and venereal disease, surgical history such as orchidopexy, inguinal hernia repair or vasectomy, current medical illness, drug history

Table 8.1: Changes in thyroid function during pregnancy

Thyroid function test	Change	Physiological cause
Total T_4 and T_3	Increased	Oestrogen-induced rise in T_4-binding globulin
Free T_4 and T_3	Increased in first trimester Decreased within normal range in second and third trimesters	High hCG concentrations in the first trimester stimulate the TSH receptor Reduction in second and third trimesters may be due to interaction of oestrogen, thyroid-binding proteins and TSH
TSH	Partial suppression in first trimester, usually within the normal range	High first-trimester hCG concentration

hCG, human chorionic gonadotrophin; T_3, triiodothyronine; T_4, thyroxine; TSH, thyroid-stimulating hormone.

replacement, antiemetics, electrolyte monitoring and vitamin supplementation (as Wernicke encephalopathy is a risk). Thyroid dysfunction does not usually need treatment, because the biochemical abnormalities resolve as the condition improves. However, a detailed history and examination should be undertaken for each patient, together with measurement of TSH receptor antibodies, because Graves' disease can present in a similar fashion. Repeat testing of thyroid function following resolution of hyperemesis is also mandatory to ensure normalization.

Optimal medical control of thyrotoxicosis in pregnancy is critical, because poorly regulated disease may be associated with:

- thyroid storm
- congestive heart failure
- an increased risk of pre-eclampsia.

Fetal health can also be compromised, with a higher incidence of:

- prematurity
- intrauterine growth restriction
- stillbirth
- congenital abnormalities.

Prior to conception, it is our practice for patients with Graves' hyperthyroidism receiving carbimazole to be changed to propylthiouracil (PTU) because of the rare reports of aplasia cutis associated with the former drug. Similarly, PTU is the drug of choice for patients presenting with thyrotoxicosis in pregnancy. Antithyroid drugs cross the placenta, and doses should be reduced as rapidly as possible to minimize the risks of fetal hypothyroidism or goitre. In practice, PTU is given in a starting dose of 100–150 mg three times daily until euthyroidism is achieved, at which time the dose is reduced to maintain clinical euthyroidism and a free T_4 concentration at the upper limit of normal. It is often possible to stop antithyroid medication altogether, as Graves' disease usually remits in the second half of pregnancy. Block and replace regimens are not suitable for use in pregnancy, because T_4 does not cross the placenta appreciably and the high doses of thionamide used increase the risk of fetal hypothyroidism. PTU enters breast milk less readily than carbimazole, and women taking PTU can therefore breast feed safely without significant risk to the neonate. However, breast feeding is not precluded in patients taking carbimazole, provided that the minimal effective dose is used and neonatal development is monitored closely. A summary of the important principles of management for Graves' hyperthyroidism in pregnancy is outlined in Figure 8.1.

Patients who are intolerant of medical therapy or who display a large goitre with pressure effects may be offered surgery as an alternative, ideally in the second trimester when the risks of spontaneous abortion are less than in early pregnancy. Radioiodine is absolutely contraindicated in pregnancy, although reports have described some cases of inappropriate administration in the face of denial of pregnancy. In these circumstances, later gestational age seems to have an adverse effect on outcome, as the fetal thyroid begins to concentrate iodine after 10–12 weeks' gestation.

On occasion, stimulating TSH receptor antibodies can cross the placenta and induce fetal or neonatal hyperthyroidism and/or goitrogenesis. Recent guidelines have clarified when and in whom TSH receptor antibodies should be measured (Table 8.2). Euthyroid women with a history of Graves' disease treated previously with antithyroid drugs alone need not have antibody measurements performed routinely, as maternal thyroid status reliably predicts fetal thyroid activity in these circumstances. In euthyroid pregnant women with previous Graves' disease treated with surgery or radioiodine therapy, TSH receptor antibodies should be checked in early pregnancy, with close fetal evaluation if a high antibody titre is evident. Antibody titres should be repeated in the last trimester. TSH receptor antibodies should also be measured at this time point in women receiving antithyroid drugs for Graves' disease during a current pregnancy. If antibody levels are high in the third trimester (Table 8.2), close involvement of an obstetrician and paediatrician is essential to monitor for fetal and neonatal thyrotoxicosis.

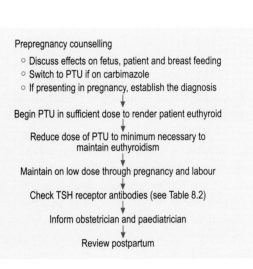

Prepregnancy counselling

- Discuss effects on fetus, patient and breast feeding
- Switch to PTU if on carbimazole
- If presenting in pregnancy, establish the diagnosis

↓

Begin PTU in sufficient dose to render patient euthyroid

↓

Reduce dose of PTU to minimum necessary to maintain euthyroidism

↓

Maintain on low dose through pregnancy and labour

↓

Check TSH receptor antibodies (see Table 8.2)

↓

Inform obstetrician and paediatrician

↓

Review postpartum

Figure 8.1
Management of Graves' thyrotoxicosis in pregnancy. Thyroid function should be monitored every 4–6 weeks. PTU, propylthiouracil; TSH, thyroid-stimulating hormone.

Table 8.2: Guidelines for thyroid-stimulating hormone receptor antibody measurement in pregnancy

Clinical status of patient	Recommendation
Euthyroid with previous medical therapy alone for Graves' disease	Measure thyroid function only.
Euthyroid with previous radioiodine therapy or surgery for Graves' disease	Measure TSH receptor antibodies[a] in early pregnancy. If antibodies undetectable or low, no further testing indicated. If antibodies high,[a] monitor fetus for hyperthyroidism and repeat TSH receptor antibodies in last trimester.
Taking antithyroid drugs for Graves' disease to maintain euthyroidism	Measure TSH receptor antibodies in last trimester. If low or undetectable, low risk of neonatal hyperthyroidism. If high,[a] evaluate neonate for hyperthyroidism.

TSH, thyroid-stimulating hormone.
[a]Specific assays measuring TSH receptor *stimulating* antibodies are useful, although most centres rely on measurement by competitive inhibition, which does not necessarily identify antibodies that are stimulating the thyroid. A commonly used method is the TRAK assay (Brahms, Berlin, Germany). With this assay, TSH receptor antibody levels above 40 U/L increase the risk of neonatal hyperthyroidism.
(After Laurberg et al. 1998, with permission.)

Hypothyroidism

Maternal hypothyroidism affects up to 2.5% of pregnancies and is most commonly due to Hashimoto's thyroiditis. The adverse effects of untreated hypothyroidism on the mother and fetus are well described, with an increased risk of spontaneous abortion, fetal abnormalities and obstetric complications. In women already taking T_4, dose requirements increase during pregnancy as evidenced by a rise in maternal TSH, patients typically needing an extra 50–100 µg of T_4 per day. The potential importance of this is highlighted by studies examining neurointellectual development in the offspring of untreated hypothyroid mothers, in which a significant reduction in childhood IQ was apparent compared with in matched control subjects. These effects are seen even in iodine-sufficient areas, raising a case for population-wide thyroid screening in early pregnancy.

Postpartum thyroid disease

Up to 10% of women develop postpartum thyroid disease, although the mild symptoms and transient nature of the syndrome in many patients mean that relatively few cases come to light. The condition is characterized by two phases: transient hyperthyroidism presenting at around 14 weeks' postpartum, followed by hypothyroidism at a later stage (median 19 weeks). Hypothyroidism is transient in the majority, although it persists in up to 30% of women or even 50% with longer term follow-up. The disease is often but not invariably associated with anti-thyroid peroxidase antibody positivity, and patients display a high risk of recurrent disease in subsequent pregnancies. In cases of doubt, the thyrotoxic phase of postpartum thyroiditis can be distinguished from Graves' disease by low uptake on a radioiodine scan and the absence of circulating TSH receptor antibodies, and from subacute thyroiditis by the absence of fever, neck tenderness or an inflammatory response.

PARATHYROID DISEASE IN PREGNANCY

Primary hyperparathyroidism

Although uncommon, primary hyperparathyroidism during pregnancy can be associated with severe maternal and perinatal complications if unrecognized or left untreated. Specific complications in pregnancy include spontaneous abortion, low birth weight and neonatal tetany (because of a functional hypoparathyroid state in the neonate consequent on fetal parathyroid suppression from transplacental passage of high maternal calcium levels). Many patients with mild disease need monitoring only, but parathyroidectomy, ideally in the second trimester, may be necessary in patients with significant hypercalcaemia.

Hypercalcaemic crisis, characterized by progressive anorexia, nausea, weakness, dehydration and stupor, can be fatal and warrants emergency treatment with adequate rehydration in the first instance. Furosemide may be added to increase urinary calcium excretion, although bisphosphonates are not recommended as their safety in pregnancy has not been established. Patients who do not respond adequately may need urgent parathyroidectomy.

PITUITARY DISEASE IN PREGNANCY

Prolactinoma

Prolactinomas are the commonest pituitary tumours and present unique challenges during pregnancy. Most are diagnosed prior to conception, and in these circumstances it is our practice to use bromocriptine in preference to cabergoline as the dopamine agonist of choice, as the safety data in pregnancy are more extensive for bromocriptine. Bromocriptine does not seem to be teratogenic, is not associated with increased incidence of spontaneous abortion or ectopic pregnancy, and long-term follow-up of the offspring of mothers treated with bromocriptine during pregnancy has not identified any developmental abnormalities. However, bromocriptine does cross the placenta and should not be used for any longer than necessary. There is considerably less experience with cabergoline, although in the smaller number of cases studied thus far it appears to be safe.

The mitogenic effects of the hyperoestrogenic environment of pregnancy on lactotroph proliferation may result in significant tumour enlargement. In this context, it is important to make the distinction between microprolactinomas (<10 mm) and macroprolactinomas (>10 mm), in which the risks are quite different. Fewer than 2% of microprolactinomas undergo clinically significant expansion, and women can safely discontinue bromocriptine once pregnancy is confirmed. The proportion of macroprolactinomas that undergo clinically relevant expansion is variable and may depend on whether tumours have been pretreated or not (26% expansion in those with no prior surgery or irradiation versus 3% in those treated with surgery or irradiation prior to pregnancy). However, in the modern era few macroprolactinomas are operated on because of the impressive efficacy of dopamine agonist therapy, and true rates of expansion in these circumstances remain unclear. Nevertheless, it would seem prudent to optimize tumour shrinkage with dopamine agonists prior to conception, with consideration being given to surgical debulking if necessary in instances in which chiasmal compression remains a concern. Bromocriptine can be discontinued in patients whose adenomas are confined to the sella but may need to be continued in patients with significant suprasellar extension. In either case, close monitoring during pregnancy is paramount and formal visual field testing should be performed every 3 months, or more frequently if signs of tumour enlargement or visual compromise are apparent. Under these circumstances, a magnetic resonance imaging (MRI) scan should be repeated. If tumour expansion does occur during pregnancy, bromocriptine should be reinstituted and visual fields followed closely in the first few days. In the unusual instance in which shrinkage does not occur or ongoing visual disturbance is apparent, surgery should be undertaken.

Prolactin levels need not be monitored during pregnancy, as they are markedly elevated (4000–6000 mU/L in the third trimester) and do not correlate with tumour activity or expansion. It is also worth noting that visual field defects have been reported in normal pregnancy, secondary to pituitary enlargement from physiological lactotroph hyperplasia.

Acromegaly

There are relatively few reports of pregnancy outcome in acromegaly because of its rarity and association with subfertility. As in the non-pregnant state, patients have an increased risk of diabetes and hypertension, but any effect of pregnancy on the extent of these complications is unclear. Maternal growth hormone does not cross the placenta and fetal outcome appears to be good in the majority of pregnancies, although some reports have demonstrated fetal growth acceleration or restriction. Tumour enlargement is uncommon, but this should be monitored as with macroprolactinomas. If tumour recurrence or expansion is apparent, bromocriptine, which is known to be safe in pregnancy, could be used, although it is effective in only a small proportion of tumours. Octreotide crosses the placenta and, in view of the widespread distribution of somatostatin receptors in the fetus and limited data regarding its safety in pregnancy, its use cannot be recommended. Pituitary surgery may be undertaken in cases in which bromocriptine is ineffective and visual function is compromised, although omitting medical therapy altogether for the duration of pregnancy is an option if sight is not threatened, given the chronic nature of the disease in the majority of patients.

Diabetes insipidus

Pregnancy alters the metabolism of vasopressin via increased glomerular filtration, enhanced placental vasopressinase activity, and induced resistance to vasopressin by increased renal prostaglandin production. These mechanisms account for the frequent observation that established diabetes insipidus may deteriorate during pregnancy, often requiring adjustment of desmopressin (DDAVP) dose. Transient cases of cranial diabetes insipidus presenting in pregnancy and resolving postpartum are also well described and attributable to these mechanisms. Simultaneous reversible loss of the posterior pituitary bright spot on T_1-weighted MRI, because of depletion of neurosecretory granules, is often seen (Fig. 8.2). Diagnosis should be based on inadequate ability to concentrate urine during a water deprivation test, although prolonged fluid restriction should be avoided. MRI of the pituitary and infundibulum should be performed in all confirmed cases and the range of causes matches those in the non-pregnant state, although lymphocytic hypophysitis has a particular predilection for pregnancy and the puerperium (see below). Desmopressin is the treatment of choice, as it exhibits markedly less oxytocic action than arginine vasopressin, with a single nocturnal dose of 10–20 µg often being sufficient. Ongoing requirements should be reviewed in the postnatal period.

Lymphocytic hypophysitis

Most cases of pregnancy-associated lymphocytic hypophysitis occur in the third trimester or puerperium and typically present with symptoms of an enlarging pituitary mass, including headaches and visual impairment. In contrast to cases presenting outside pregnancy, symptoms of hypopituitarism are often minimal or absent. However, investigations usually demonstrate a variable degree of hypopituitarism, with a predilection for adrenocorticotrophic hormone (ACTH) and/or TSH deficiency. Diabetes insipidus is present in up to 10% and may help differentiate hypophysitis from pituitary adenoma, but this is not absolute. Although management is contentious, a conservative approach is generally favoured in pregnancy provided that patients are monitored closely, with frequent assessment of visual fields and pituitary function. Following delivery, evaluation should also include repeat MRI scans. Most cases in pregnancy resolve spontaneously, but recovery of pituitary function may be unrelated to change in size of the pituitary mass.

Hypopituitarism

Although pregnancy is more difficult to achieve in patients with hypopituitarism (usually requiring ovulation induction), adjustment of medication may be important. Growth hormone replacement should be discontinued because of inadequate safety information on its use in pregnancy and lactation. Thyroid hormone levels may need to be increased as in primary hypothyroidism. Glucocorticoid replacement doses may also need to be increased in some symptomatic patients in the third trimester to mimic the physiological rise in cortisol-binding globulin and free cortisol, although in practice this is rarely necessary. All patients need high-dose parenteral glucocorticoid replacement during labour, with rapid tailing of the dose to prepregnancy levels in the puerperium. Hypopituitarism occasionally presents for the first time during pregnancy and is usually due to lymphocytic hypophysitis. Hypopituitarism arising postpartum is usually

Treatment of adrenal Cushing's syndrome involves adrenalectomy, which should not be delayed because of a higher risk of malignant disease (over 20%) in pregnancy, although in patients presenting late in their third trimester early delivery prior to definitive therapy may be considered.

Addison's disease

Primary adrenal insufficiency rarely presents during pregnancy, but its presence should be considered in any pregnant woman with:

- prolonged nausea
- weight loss
- hypotension
- syncope
- weakness
- characteristic electrolyte disturbance.

Establishment of the diagnosis is as in the non-pregnant state (see Ch. 5), although allowances need to be made for the physiological changes that occur in the hypothalamic–pituitary–adrenal axis. Hydrocortisone replacement may need to be increased in the third trimester to mimic the physiological rise in cortisol at this stage, and the mineralocorticoid dose may need adjustment according to blood pressure and electrolyte status, as the increase in serum progesterone exerts an antimineralocorticoid action. Plasma renin activity cannot be used for monitoring because of a physiological increase during pregnancy. Labour and obstetric emergency should be covered with high-dose parenteral steroid replacement together with intravenous fluids if necessary.

Congenital adrenal hyperplasia

Advances in genital reconstructive surgery, better compliance with replacement therapy, and earlier treatment of congenital adrenal hyperplasia (CAH) have contributed to improved fertility in this condition. In women with CAH, hydrocortisone or prednisolone should be used as the glucocorticoid replacement therapy of choice, as they are metabolized by the placenta and do not affect fetal hypothalamic–pituitary–adrenal axis activity. Dexamethasone is able to cross the placenta and should not be used as replacement therapy in women with CAH, although it is used therapeutically in pregnancies in which the fetus may be at risk of developing CAH (e.g. in a woman with CAH whose partner is a carrier; see below).

Monitoring of treatment in pregnancy should include periodic measurement of testosterone in addition to 17-hydroxyprogesterone, as the latter rises during pregnancy and may be unreliable when used alone, especially in early pregnancy, when adequate suppression of testosterone is most important. The glucocorticoid doses used should be sufficient to keep maternal testosterone levels at the upper end of the normal reference range. Glucocorticoid requirements may increase in the third trimester and, as with any patient with suppression of the hypothalamic–pituitary–adrenal axis, labour should be covered with high-dose parenteral steroids. Patients who have previously undergone genital reconstructive surgery should undergo elective caesarean section to minimize trauma to the genital tract.

Women with CAH are not unreasonably concerned regarding the chances of their child inheriting the condition, although the actual risk of having an affected fetus is low. The population carrier rate varies from one in 17 to one in 50, meaning that women with CAH have a one in 68 to one in 200 chance of having an affected female, rising to one in 4 if their partner is a carrier. Women with CAH who are planning pregnancy should therefore undergo careful preconception genetic counselling with testing of carrier status in the partner.

Maternal therapy with dexamethasone has been advocated for fetuses at risk for CAH, and it is clear that very early treatment significantly reduces virilization in affected females, although the extent of this is variable. There are no consistent adverse effects of this strategy on fetal outcome in utero, and birth weight is not reduced. Furthermore, despite potential concerns regarding the safety of steroid administration on the developing fetal brain, follow-up studies on small numbers of children treated in this manner – whether treated to term or in the seven of eight fetuses in whom therapy is stopped because of heterozygosity, male sex or being unaffected – have not revealed cognitive or motor deficits to date. Continued vigilance is essential, however, as few treated fetuses have reached adulthood. Mothers treated with dexamethasone gain weight and develop oedema but do not seem to be at a greater risk of developing hypertension or gestational diabetes.

A recent consensus statement has outlined the criteria for prenatal treatment in CAH. These include:

- confirmation by DNA analysis of a previously affected sibling or first-degree relative with known mutations causing classic CAH
- availability of rapid, reliable genetic testing
- early institution of therapy after the last menstrual period.

Dexamethasone should be administered at a dose of 20 µg/kg of maternal body weight per day in three divided doses and should be commenced as soon as pregnancy is confirmed and no later than 9 weeks' gestation. Chorionic villus biopsy should be performed at 10–12 weeks' gestation and treatment continued to term in affected female fetuses only. This approach will evidently result in unnecessary treatment in seven out of eight fetuses (because CAH is inherited as an autosomal recessive disease and only affected girls benefit from treatment), highlighting the need for meticulous preconception counselling and prospective follow-up of all children treated in this manner. Registries for children who received prenatal dexamethasone are being encouraged to address this issue. A summary of the prenatal diagnosis and treatment of fetuses at risk of CAH is shown in Figure 8.3.

Primary hyperaldosteronism

There are very few cases of Conn's syndrome reported in pregnancy, and most patients will have been diagnosed prior to conception. Spironolactone, which is often used in

Figure 8.3
Prenatal treatment of fetuses at risk of congenital adrenal hyperplasia (previous child with congenital adrenal hyperplasia or affected mother and carrier father).

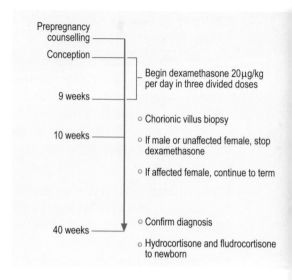

treating this condition, can cross the placenta and may cause abnormal genital development because of its antiandrogenic properties. Spironolactone should therefore be discontinued prior to conception if possible and the hypertension controlled by other antihypertensive agents used in pregnancy, such as methyldopa, nifedipine or labetalol. Surgery may be necessary if medical therapy fails to adequately control the hypertension.

Phaeochromocytoma

Phaeochromocytoma presents rarely during pregnancy, but it is an important condition to diagnose because of the significant adverse effects on the fetus and the mother in untreated disease. Historically, maternal mortality approached 50%, but early diagnosis, optimal predelivery adrenergic blockade and appropriate multidisciplinary delivery strategies have reduced this significantly. Nevertheless, a recent *Report on Confidential Enquiries into Maternal Deaths in the United Kingdom* recorded five deaths caused by unrecognized phaeochromocytoma, highlighting the need for continued vigilance.

Given that early pharmacological intervention improves outcome, it is clearly imperative to establish the diagnosis as soon as possible. In patients at high risk – such as those with a personal or family history of multiple endocrine neoplasia type 2, von Hippel–Lindau syndrome (VHL), neurofibromatosis type 1 or hereditary paraganglioma syndrome (from germline mutations in subunits of the mitochondrial enzyme succinate dehydrogenase) – screening with 24-h urinary fractionated metanephrines or free catecholamine measurement as in the non-pregnant state should take place not only prior to conception but also during pregnancy, especially in individuals whose particular gene mutation places them at notably higher risk (e.g. missesnse mutations in the VHL gene).

Diagnosis of sporadic cases presenting in pregnancy is often difficult, although a high index of suspicion should be maintained in:

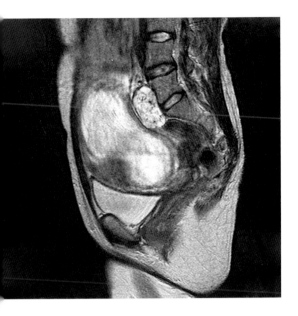

Figure 8.4
Magnetic resonance imaging scan of paraganglioma
(organ of Zuckerkandl) in a 32-year-old primigravida
identified with hypertension in the first trimester (scan
performed at 18 weeks' gestation). Following
preoperative preparation with phenoxybenzamine and
atenolol, she underwent a successful laparotomy to
remove the tumour at 22 weeks.

- women with severe or early-onset hypertension
- women with wide fluctuations in blood pressure or with glycosuria
- those describing paroxysms of pallor, palpitations, headache or sweating.

Following confirmation of the diagnosis by a finding of elevated catecholamines in a 24-h urine collection, MRI should be used for tumour localization (Fig. 8.4), because computerized tomography and metaiodobenzylguanidine scans are contraindicated in pregnancy due to the radiation involved.

Management centres on alpha blockade with phenoxybenzamine followed by beta blockade to regulate tachycardia. Phenoxybenzamine is safe in pregnancy and, although beta blockers are associated with intrauterine growth restriction, such concerns are usually outweighed by the need for adequate treatment of the tumour. Surgery is the mainstay of subsequent therapy, although controversy remains about its timing. Most authors recommend surgical removal in patients whose tumours have been identified before 24 weeks' gestation. Concerns relating to difficult surgical access beyond 24 weeks would lead many to delay surgery in the remainder until fetal maturity is reached at 34 weeks' gestation or more. Surgical resection is then combined with caesarean section at this stage or performed at a later date. Caesarean section is the preferred mode of delivery because of concerns relating to pressure on the tumour from uterine contractions. However, spontaneous vaginal delivery has been reported to pass uneventfully in carefully selected patients with optimal predelivery blockade.

Further reading

Bronstein MD (ed.) 2001 Pituitary tumors and pregnancy. Kluwer, Norwell
de Swiet M 1995 Diseases of the pituitary and adrenal gland. In: de Swiet M (ed.) Medical disorders in obstetric practice, 3rd edn. Blackwell, Oxford, pp. 483–504

Joint Lawson Wilkins Pediatric Endocrine Society–European Society for Paediatric Endocrinology Congenital Adrenal Hyperplasia Working Group 2002 Consensus statement on 21-hydroxylase deficiency from the Lawson Wilkins Pediatric Endocrine Society and the European Society for Paediatric Endocrinology. J Clin Endocrinol Metab 87: 4048–4053

Laurberg P, Nygaard B, Glinoer D et al. 1998 Guidelines for TSH-receptor antibody measurements in pregnancy: results of an evidence-based symposium organized by the European Thyroid Association. Eur J Endocrinol 139: 584–590

Lazarus JH, Kokandi A 2000 Thyroid disease in relation to pregnancy: a decade of change. Clin Endocrinol 53: 265–278

SELF-ASSESSMENT

Patient 1

A 22-year-old lady, in her third pregnancy, presents to her local hospital at 35 weeks' gestation with modest hypertension (blood pressure 130/90 mmHg). She is known to carry a mutation for VHL but has had no prior disease manifestations and her previous pregnancies have passed uneventfully, resulting in spontaneous vaginal delivery of two healthy children. Her 24-h urinary catecholamine levels are within normal limits at 18 weeks' gestation, and she has remained asymptomatic throughout her pregnancy.

Questions
1. What investigations should she have?
2. How should she be treated?

Answers
1. The patient is at high risk of developing a phaeochromocytoma, and 24-h urinary fractionated metanephrines or free catecholamines should be measured, proceeding to MRI of the adrenals if these values are elevated. A careful clinical assessment should also be performed for other complications of VHL, including detailed neurological examination (with or without MRI of the brain and spinal cord if indicated), fundoscopy (for retinal angiomas) and urinalysis.

   The noradrenaline (norepinephrine) and normetadrenaline (normetanephrine) values were elevated on repeat testing (1761 nmol/24 h and 9.69 μmol/24 h, respectively; normal ranges 60–660 nmol/24 h and <4 μmol/24 h), and MRI demonstrated the presence of a 2.5-cm right-sided adrenal mass (Fig. 8.5). MRI of the brain and spinal cord did not reveal other disease manifestations of VHL.

2. Once a diagnosis of phaeochromocytoma is established, the patient should be commenced on phenoxybenzamine, titrating the dose upwards according to postural blood pressure measurements. Beta blockade should then be instituted to control tachycardia. Optimal delivery and operative strategy require a multidisciplinary approach involving an endocrinologist, anaesthetist with experience in managing phaeochromocytoma, obstetrician and endocrine surgeon. Elective caesarean section should be recommended as the preferred mode of delivery and can be combined with adrenalectomy. Alternatively, adrenalectomy may be delayed until 6 weeks after delivery. Intravenous phentolamine should be available for any hypertensive crisis, although recent reports also point to the effectiveness of magnesium in this setting.

   Subsequent management should include triennial surveillance MRI of the brain and abdomen, and annual fundoscopy, urinalysis and 24-h urine collections for fractionated metanephrines or free catecholamines. Genetic testing for a VHL mutation in her child should also be performed.

Figure 8.5
Abdominal magnetic resonance imaging scan demonstrating 2.5-cm right adrenal mass.

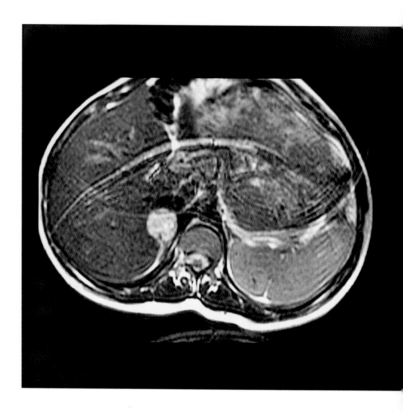

Patient 2

A 23-year-old lady, in her first pregnancy, presents to her obstetrician with a history of peripheral and facial oedema. Her previous medical and family history is unremarkable. The current pregnancy is complicated by a diagnosis of gestational diabetes at 20 weeks, rapidly requiring treatment with significant doses of insulin. Examination reveals peripheral oedema, acneform rash over the trunk, hypertension (blood pressure 150/80 mmHg, blood pressure at booking visit 110/70 mmHg), +4 glycosuria on dipstick urinalysis and purple striae as shown in Figure 8.6. Ultrasound examination reveals a healthy fetus and placenta but a diffuse hyperechoic pattern within the liver, consistent with fatty change.

Questions
1. What is the diagnosis and which investigations should be performed to confirm this?
2. How should she be treated?
3. What complication could ensue, and how would you avoid this?

Answers
1. The clinical findings, early-onset hypertension and early diabetes in pregnancy all suggest a diagnosis of Cushing's syndrome. Investigations should include measurement of 24-h urinary free cortisol, cortisol response to overnight dexamethasone (1 mg) proceeding to cortisol response to 48 h of low-dose dexamethasone (0.5 mg q.d.s.) if

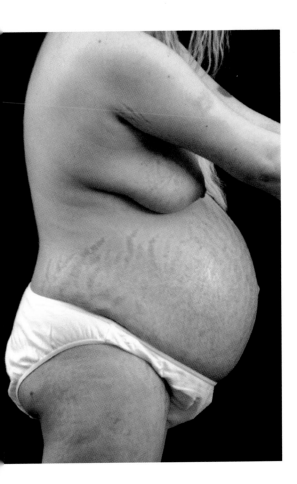

Figure 8.6
Purple striae in pregnancy.

screening tests indicate the need. Subsequent tests directed at localizing the cause should include ACTH measurement and MRI of the adrenals or pituitary as indicated. This patient had elevated 9 a.m. and midnight cortisol levels with loss of diurnal variation (1169 nmol/L at 9 a.m., 1137 nmol/L at midnight) and elevated urinary free cortisol concentration (1350 and 1297 nmol/24 h), and she failed to suppress serum cortisol below 244 nmol/L after 48 h of 0.5-mg dexamethasone. ACTH levels were undetectable, and MRI of the adrenals demonstrated a 4-cm right adrenal mass.

2. The definitive treatment is adrenalectomy, which should not be delayed. The hypertension and diabetes should be optimally controlled prior to surgery, and a laparoscopic approach, which is feasible at this gestation, would be preferred in view of possible concerns relating to poor wound healing in the postoperative period.

3. The patient is at risk of post-surgery hypocortisolism, as the contralateral adrenal gland will be suppressed. Parenteral followed by oral steroid therapy should be administered in anticipation. This should take the form of hydrocortisone (or prednisolone), as it does not cross the placenta. Adequate recovery of adrenal function in the contralateral gland may take some time and should be assessed by periodic

short synacthen tests in parallel with a decreasing glucocorticoid replacement schedule. In many cases, especially with significant hypercortisolism from large tumours, it is not feasible for patients to withdraw therapy during pregnancy; in these circumstances, it is important to increase steroid doses peridelivery. The need for ongoing steroid therapy can then be addressed in the postpartum period.

Neuroendocrine and inherited endocrine tumours

9

A. Rees

NEUROENDOCRINE TUMOURS

Neuroendocrine tumours (NETs) represent a heterogeneous group of neoplasms with significant variation in their mode of presentation and biological behaviour. They arise from neuroendocrine cells that are widely distributed in the body; the spectrum of tumours that fall into this classification is accordingly diverse and may include:

- gastroenteropancreatic NETs
- medullary carcinoma of the thyroid
- small cell carcinoma of the lung
- phaeochromocytoma.

However, this section will focus solely on gastroenteropancreatic and bronchial NETs. Although the aetiology of these tumours is poorly understood, significant advances have been made recently in their diagnosis and management, and these will be highlighted.

Epidemiology and natural history

Neuroendocrine tumours are uncommon tumours with an estimated annual incidence of three per 100 000. The natural history of NETs varies according to the site of the primary tumour and stage at presentation (Fig. 9.1); recent data suggest that survival may be improving. Pancreatic NETs are particularly rare, with an annual incidence of 0.1–1 per million, non-functioning tumours being the commonest. Prognosis is closely related to tumour phenotype, with malignancy being uncommon in insulinomas (Table 9.1).

Genetic testing

A small proportion of NETs have a familial basis, and clinical evaluation should include a detailed family history and examination to search for features of multiple endocrine neoplasia type 1 (MEN-1) or type 2 (MEN-2), von Hippel–Lindau syndrome (VHL), neurofibromatosis type 1 (NF-1) and Carney complex (see p. 228) as appropriate. Genetic testing is now widely available for most of these conditions, and molecular analysis of the relevant gene should be undertaken if there is a positive family history or

Figure 9.1
Average 5-year survival rates in bronchial, gastric and intestinal neuroendocrine tumours according to site of primary tumour and stage at presentation.

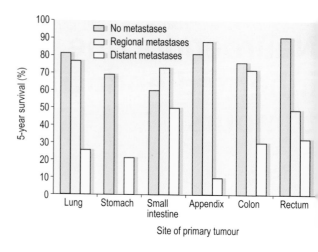

Table 9.1: Epidemiology and incidence of malignancy at presentation in pancreatic neuroendocrine tumours

Tumour type	Annual incidence	Malignancy (%)
Insulinoma	1–2 per million	<10
Gastrinoma	1 per million	>50
Vasoactive intestinal peptide-producing tumour (VIPoma)	1 per 5 million	>50
Glucagonoma	1 per 5 million	>70
Pancreatic polypeptideoma	1 per 10 million	>60
Somatostatinoma	1 per 10 million	>50

a second endocrine tumour, not only for confirmation of the diagnosis and rationalization of management in the affected patient, but also to enable presymptomatic testing in relatives. In particular, a potential diagnosis of MEN-1 should be considered in patients with bronchial or gastric carcinoid tumours, or in cases of gastrinoma or multiple islet cell tumours (Box 9.1). In addition, a small familial clustering of midgut and hindgut NETs is recognized that is independent of MEN-1.

Clinical presentation

In keeping with the widespread distribution of these tumours, their modes of presentation vary considerably. Many are discovered incidentally as part of investigation for other reasons (e.g. at endoscopy or colonoscopy) or present with intestinal obstruction. Classic carcinoid syndrome is a presenting feature in less than 10% of patients and occurs when vasogenic amines and peptides, including serotonin, gain access to the systemic circulation. It is usually seen in the context of metastatic NETs of embryological midgut origin (small intestine, appendix, right colon). The main features of classic carcinoid syndrome are flushing (90%) and diarrhoea (70%), with abdominal pain (40%), valvular heart disease (40%), wheezing (25%) and pellagra (5%) occurring

Box 9.1: Indications for multiple endocrine neoplasia type 1 mutational analysis

In an index case

- Case meets criteria for sporadic multiple endocrine neoplasia type 1 (MEN-1) (presence of at least two out of the three main MEN-1-related tumours: parathyroid, pituitary, pancreatic)
- Case meets criteria for familial MEN-1 (as in sporadic MEN-1 plus at least one first-degree relative with one of the three principal MEN-1-related tumours)
- Suspicious/atypical of MEN-1 (two or more MEN-1-related tumours, multiple parathyroid tumours before age 30, recurrent hyperparathyroidism, gastrinoma or multiple islet cell tumours, familial isolated hyperparathyroidism)

In member of family with known MEN-1 mutation

- Asymptomatic relative
- Relative expressing familial MEN-1

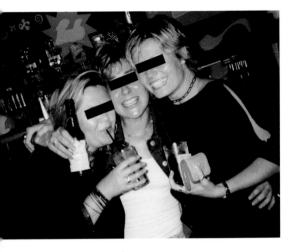

Figure 9.2
A facial flush in a patient with medullary thyroid carcinoma.

less frequently. The carcinoid flush is usually pink, lasts for a few minutes and involves the face and upper trunk. Some patients are able to identify triggers such as alcohol, bananas, walnuts or chocolate. Atypical carcinoid syndrome is occasionally seen in a small proportion of patients with foregut carcinoid tumours and consists of a protracted purplish flush leaving cutaneous telangiectasia in the face, upper trunk and limbs, although a fixed facial flush may also develop in patients with long-standing classic carcinoid syndrome. Other causes of flushing, such as medullary thyroid carcinoma (MTC; Fig. 9.2), are listed in Table 9.2.

Carcinoid crisis is an extreme presentation and is life-threatening. Characterized by hypotension, tachycardia/arrhythmias, flushing, wheezing and nervous system disturbance, it may be precipitated by tumour lysis (from embolization, chemotherapy or radionuclide therapy), tumour handling or anaesthesia, and it necessitates urgent treatment with octreotide infusion.

Bronchial NETs may present with symptoms suggestive of bronchial obstruction (pneumonia, dyspnoea, pleuritic pain), cough or haemoptysis, although many tumours

Table 9.2: Causes of flushing

Condition	Associated clinical features
Carcinoid syndrome	Diarrhoea, wheeze, valvular heart disease
Medullary thyroid carcinoma	Mass in neck, diarrhoea, possible family history
Menopause	Cessation of menses, mood change, vaginal dryness, loss of libido
Phaeochromocytoma	Hypertension, headache, palpitations
Diabetes	Secondary to autonomic neuropathy or chlorpropamide
Panic attacks	Anxiety, hyperventilation, phobias
Mastocytosis	Urticaria pigmentosa, dermatographia, dyspepsia, peptic ulcer
Drugs	Nicotinic acid, acipimox, calcium channel blockers, chlorpropamide
Autonomic epilepsy	Diencephalic seizures
Idiopathic	–

Table 9.3: Clinical syndromes in enteropancreatic neuroendocrine tumours

Tumour type	Symptoms
Insulinoma	Neuroglycopenia, weight gain
Gastrinoma	Peptic ulceration, diarrhoea
Glucagonoma	Diabetes, weight loss, necrolytic migratory erythema
Vasoactive intestinal peptide-producing tumour (VIPoma)	Watery diarrhoea, severe hypokalaemia
Somatostatinoma	Steatorrhoea, cholelithiasis, weight loss, diabetes

do not cause symptoms and are discovered incidentally on a chest x-ray. Bronchial NETs may also cause ectopic hormone production (e.g. Cushing's syndrome from ectopic adrenocorticotrophic hormone, acromegaly from ectopic growth hormone-releasing hormone, or the syndrome of inappropriate antidiuretic hormone secretion, SIADH).

Pancreatic NETs present either with a hypersecretory syndrome (Table 9.3) or with symptoms due to tumour mass effect or metastases.

Carcinoid heart disease is characterized by thickened deposits in the endocardium, classically affecting the right side of the heart in patients with carcinoid syndrome, with tricuspid regurgitation being the most common valvular lesion. The cause of the condition is unclear, but a recent study has suggested that progression of valvular disease may be greater in patients who have received cytotoxic chemotherapy or who have rising urinary 5-hydroxyindoleacetic acid (5-HIAA) concentrations. Right-sided heart disease is associated with substantial morbidity and mortality such that a significant proportion of patients with carcinoid syndrome die of carcinoid heart disease rather than from tumour growth. Accordingly, valve replacement surgery should be considered in all patients whose disease elsewhere is controllable. At present, it seems that somatostatin analogue therapy does not prevent disease progression, although it is not known whether therapy prevents disease development.

Diagnosis

Biochemical testing

Blood and urine measurements are useful in the management of NETs, not only as an aid to diagnosis but also in establishing prognosis and in monitoring response to treatment. Plasma chromogranin A (CgA) is a useful general tumour marker and retains high sensitivity (70–90%) in most types of NET, with the highest levels often seen in metastatic midgut NETs. Renal impairment and hypergastrinaemia are important causes of false positive CgA elevation. CgA may additionally have prognostic relevance for midgut NETs, as it correlates with tumour load and biological activity. Patients with midgut NETs also secrete serotonin, although plasma measurement of this peptide is usually replaced by urinary measurement of its metabolite 5-HIAA. Urinary 5-HIAA shows high sensitivity (70%) in midgut carcinoid disease but is generally not raised in patients with foregut or hindgut tumours. A number of foodstuffs and drugs can affect interpretation of results (Box 9.2), although these are rarely problematic in clinical practice.

Tachykinins such as neurokinin A are showing promise as good prognostic markers and in evaluating response to treatment in midgut NETs. However, levels are not elevated in all patients, and analysis is currently available in research laboratories only. Other biochemical markers may be useful in diagnosis, depending on the clinical presentation (e.g. α-human chorionic gonadotrophin for hindgut tumours) and the index of suspicion for inherited disease (e.g. prolactin, calcium, parathyroid hormone if MEN-1 is suspected). A fasting gut hormone profile should complement plasma CgA measurement in suspected pancreatic NETs. Blood should be collected into a lithium heparin bottle containing Trasylol, spun, and frozen prior to analysis at one of the two reference

---

Box 9.2: Substances affecting interpretation of urinary 5-hydroxyindoleacetic acid measurement

False positive

- Aubergine
- Avocado
- Banana
- Caffeine
- Fluorouracil
- Methysergide
- Naproxen
- Paracetamol (acetaminophen)
- Pineapple
- Plums
- Walnut

False negative

- Adrenocorticotrophic hormone
- Aspirin
- Levodopa
- Methyldopa
- Phenothiazines

laboratories currently in the UK (Peptide Laboratory, Hammersmith Hospital, London; Regional Regulatory Peptide Laboratory, Royal Victoria Hospital, Belfast). Currently, gastrin, glucagon, somatostatin, vasointestinal peptide, pancreatic polypeptide and neurotensin are measured. It is important to remember that patients should be off proton pump inhibitors for 2 weeks and off H_2 inhibitors for at least 3 days to avoid false positive gastrin measurements.

Patients with insulinomas usually present with symptoms of hypoglycaemia. These may be non-specific (unexplained collapse, 'funny turn') or more classically adrenergic (pallor, perspiration, tachycardia) or neuroglycopenic (irritability, change in behaviour, confusion, seizures, coma). If spontaneous hypoglycaemia from a possible insulinoma is suspected, a prolonged 72-h fast is the investigation of choice, detecting 98% of patients with insulinoma. Shorter duration fasts have lower sensitivity (75% and 90–94% at 24 and 48 h, respectively). Patients are allowed to drink water freely and should have plasma glucose, proinsulin, insulin, C-peptide and β-hydroxybutyrate levels measured daily and when they are symptomatic. Patients who fail to demonstrate hypoglycaemia (plasma glucose below 2.2 mmol/L) by the end of the fast should be exercised for 15 min. The fast is then terminated at the end of this period of exercise or when hypoglycaemia is confirmed at any stage. The biochemistry in patients harbouring an insulinoma will reveal inappropriate elevation of insulin (often with disproportionately high proinsulin) and C-peptide and suppression of β-hydroxybutyrate in the face of hypoglycaemia, although it is mandatory that plasma and urine samples are analysed simultaneously for sulphonylurea. An important practice point emerges from a recent report demonstrating 'reactive' hypoglycaemia in two patients with confirmed insulinoma; both had normal 72-h fasts but significant hyperinsulinaemia and hypoglycaemia following a prolonged oral glucose tolerance test. This emphasizes the importance of clinical judgement in the evaluation of suspected insulinoma; if the index of suspicion is high, an apparently normal 72-h fast does not necessarily exclude the diagnosis.

A summary of other causes of hypoglycaemia is shown in Box 9.3. A careful history should determine whether symptoms occur predominantly in the fasting or postprandial (2–5 h after food) state, as the initial investigations may differ (supervised fast for the former, prolonged oral glucose tolerance test for the latter). Baseline biochemical tests may also include liver function tests, alcohol concentration and cortisol (with or without synacthen) levels. Rarely, patients may require investigation for non-islet cell tumour hypoglycaemia; such patients usually have large thoracic or retroperitoneal mesenchymal tumours producing excess insulin-like growth factor (IGF)-2. Measurement of IGF-2:IGF-1 molar ratio may therefore help in the diagnosis.

Imaging

A number of imaging modalities are employed in the evaluation of NETs. Determining an appropriate imaging strategy in an individual patient will require close liaison with radiologists and nuclear medicine physicians, but it is partly dependent on whether the imaging is undertaken for initial detection of the disease in suspected cases or in determining tumour extent when neuroendocrine disease is already confirmed. In

---

Box 9.3: Causes of hypoglycaemia

Fasting hypoglycaemia

- Drugs (insulin, sulphonylureas, quinine, salicylates, alcohol)
- Hormone deficiency (adrenal insufficiency, hypopituitarism)
- Organ failure (liver failure, chronic renal failure)
- Insulinoma
- Non-islet cell tumours (fibrosarcoma, mesothelioma, hepatocellular carcinoma)
- Autoimmune (insulin receptor-activating antibodies)
- Infection (septicaemia, malaria)
- Inborn errors of metabolism (glycogen storage disease, hereditary fructose intolerance, maple syrup disease)
- β-cell hyperplasia/adult nesidioblastosis

Postprandial hypoglycaemia

- Alcohol-induced
- Incipient diabetes mellitus
- Postgastrectomy
- Idiopathic

---

searching for primary NETs, a multimodal imaging approach is often needed and may include one or more of:

- ultrasonography
- computerized tomography (CT)
- magnetic resonance imaging (MRI)
- somatostatin receptor scintigraphy (SSRS, 'octreoscan', indium-111 octreotide)
- iodine-123 metaiodobenzylguanidine (MIBG) scintigraphy
- endoscopy
- endoscopic ultrasound
- positron emission tomography (PET)
- angiography/venous sampling.

Somatostatin receptor scintigraphy has high sensitivity in locating primary NETs (70–80%) and in assessing the extent of metastatic disease (90%). The exception to this is insulinomas, for which sensitivity falls to less than 50%. Modern nuclear imaging centres now use SSRS in combination with single positron emission computed tomography and fusion imaging with CT to enhance sensitivity (Fig. 9.3). Demonstration of clear uptake on SSRS also predicts response to somatostatin analogue therapy and will determine suitability for targeted radiolabelled therapy. Iodine-123 MIBG has significantly lower sensitivity (only 50% sensitivity for metastases) than indium-111 octreotide but may also be useful when targeted radiotherapy is being considered. CT scans are useful in identifying lung NETs, in assessing liver metastases (where triple phase enhances sensitivity) and in identifying primary abdominal NETs, especially when SSRS is negative. MRI and CT are both useful in imaging pancreatic NETs, although endoscopic ultrasound is particularly sensitive, especially in identifying lesions within the pancreatic head (Fig. 9.4). Studies examining the value of PET scanning in neuroendocrine disease are still in progress, although its widespread use is currently limited by scanner

Figure 9.3
Somatostatin receptor scanning with computerized tomography colocalization.

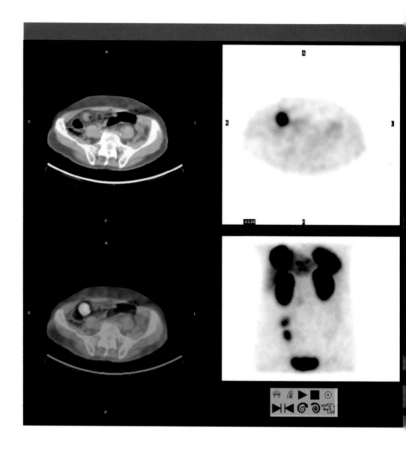

Figure 9.4
Endoscopic ultrasound appearances of an insulinoma (arrow).

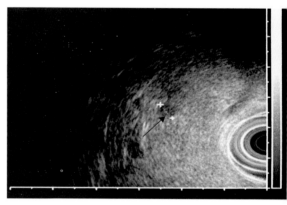

availability. However, fluorodeoxyglucose-18 PET is often negative in indolent disease; if uptake is present, this may correlate with a poorer prognosis.

There is limited experience with other tracers at present, although 18-fluorodopa and carbon-11 tryptophan are under evaluation. Selective angiography with secretagogue injection may be particularly useful in localizing small gastrinomas or insulinomas, especially when other radiology has been normal. The main pancreatic arteries (gastroduodenal, superior mesenteric, inferior pancreaticoduodenal and splenic) are cannulated and examined for a tumour blush. Calcium is injected into each artery in turn, and samples are collected for hormone measurement (for insulin or gastrin as appropriate) from the hepatic vein. A rise in the hormone level (as opposed to a fall in normal subjects) facilitates localization of the tumour and may enable biochemical distinction of multiple pancreatic tumours in MEN-1. Finally, direct palpation at laparotomy is sensitive, especially when combined with intraoperative ultrasound.

Pathology

The World Health Organization has recently revised the classification of gastroenteropancreatic NETs into four groups based on a variety of gross and microscopic features:

1. well-differentiated endocrine tumour of probable benign behaviour
2. well-differentiated endocrine tumour of uncertain behaviour
3. well-differentiated endocrine carcinoma
4. poorly differentiated endocrine carcinoma.

Immunohistochemistry using a panel of antibodies directed against general neuroendocrine markers (e.g. synaptophysin and CgA) is used to confirm a neuroendocrine source and is supplemented with immunostaining for appropriate hormones when a syndrome of hormone excess is suspected clinically (Fig. 9.5). In

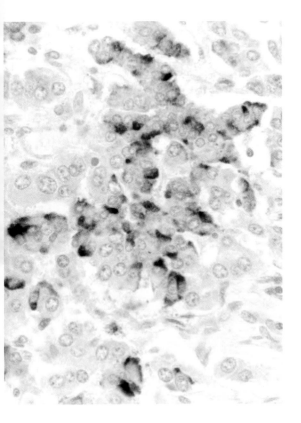

Figure 9.5
Glucagon immunostaining in a pancreatic glucagonoma.

addition, assessment of the proliferative potential of the tumour using Ki-67 staining is prognostically important, especially in pancreatic NETs, and may have some value in determining mode of therapy (e.g. chemotherapy in poorly differentiated NETs with high Ki-67 index).

Management

Because NETs are rare, there are limited randomized trial data to form a robust evidence base to guide management. Few individual units will have developed sufficient experience to confidently evaluate this diverse range of tumours, and all cases should therefore be managed in the context of a multidisciplinary team whose members will vary according to local expertise and interests but which should comprise representation from endocrinology, gastroenterology, surgery, oncology, radiology/nuclear medicine and histopathology. A multidisciplinary approach will facilitate accurate diagnosis and staging, develop consensus agreement on management, ensure individualized treatment planning and improve interdisciplinary education. Increasingly, such groups should form part of a larger network of clinicians with interests in these tumours at national (UKNETwork) and international (European Neuroendocrine Tumour Society) levels, thereby facilitating multicentre studies and development of consensus guidelines.

Surgery

Where possible, the aim of treatment is to cure the patient, and surgery is currently the only available treatment modality that can achieve this. However, metastatic disease at presentation frequently precludes surgical cure, and treatment then becomes palliative, although surgery may still have a role in debulking the primary tumour and minimizing the risk of intestinal obstruction. Preoperatively, patients with known functioning midgut NETs should be carefully assessed for the presence of carcinoid heart disease and should be treated in the pre-, peri- and postoperative periods with an intravenous infusion of octreotide (50 µg/h) in order to minimize the risk of carcinoid crisis. Patients with bronchial NETs should undergo lung or wedge resection with lymph node dissection. The surgical management of gastroenteropancreatic NETs is dependent on the primary site, mode of presentation (elective versus emergency) and extent of disease. Emergency presentations usually demand a resection sufficient to correct the immediate problem but may need to be followed by a further more definitive procedure, for example in patients presenting with appendicitis when prognosis can be improved by performing a right hemicolectomy in appendiceal tumours greater than 2 cm in size, or in lesions of 1–2 cm when the macro- or microscopic appearances are unfavourable. Small intestinal and colorectal NETs should be resected together with extensive locoregional lymph node dissection.

Gastric NETs are classified into three types.

- Type 1 gastric NETs are associated with hypergastrinaemia and chronic atrophic gastritis and have low malignant potential. They can therefore be managed by endoscopic surveillance or limited surgery (polypectomy and/or antrectomy) only.

- Type 2 gastric NETs are seen in patients with Zollinger–Ellison syndrome and MEN-1 and may be treated with proton pump inhibitors.
- Type 3 gastric NETs occur sporadically, are more aggressive and will frequently show evidence of metastasis at presentation. Most will need gastrectomy and regional lymph node clearance.

Surgery for pancreatic NETs should be performed only by pancreaticobiliary specialists, and its extent can vary from enucleation only for superficial or easily localized insulinomas (which have low malignant potential) to distal or total pancreatectomy or even pancreatoduodenectomy in more extensive disease. Liver resection of unilobar liver metastases may prolong survival and can additionally offer symptomatic relief in carefully selected cases in which a single hepatic lesion is dominant. Whenever abdominal surgery is contemplated for NETs, consideration should always be given to cholecystectomy in order to prevent gallstone formation in patients who are subsequently begun on somatostatin analogues.

Drug therapy

Somatostatin analogue therapy

Somatostatin analogue therapy forms the mainstay of symptomatic control in gastroenteropancreatic NETs. The endogenous hormone somatostatin has a very short circulatory half-life, making it unsuitable for use. Octreotide has a half-life of several hours and can be administered subcutaneously in doses of 50–100 µg two or three times daily (up to a maximum daily dose of 1500 µg). More recently, sustained-release preparations have become available, allowing dosing every 2–4 weeks.

There are three drugs in routine use:

1. lanreotide (fortnightly injection)
2. lanreotide Autogel (monthly)
3. octreotide (Sandostatin LAR) (monthly).

All these drugs have been shown to improve quality of life (including a reduction in the frequency of flushing and diarrhoea attacks), with equivalent or improved efficacy compared with short-acting octreotide. Patients are usually begun on octreotide for 1–2 weeks to assess tolerability and to enable symptom stabilization prior to conversion to a long-acting preparation. In addition to good symptomatic control, which occurs in the vast majority of patients, biochemical response occurs in 30–70% and tumour stabilization (or rarely even shrinkage) may occur. Patients should be warned to expect gastrointestinal side-effects (such as diarrhoea, abdominal discomfort, flatulence, anorexia and nausea) at the start of therapy, which are usually mild and diminish with continued use. In addition, patients with diabetes may need to adjust their insulin dose. Long-term use can result in gallstone formation, although these are rarely symptomatic, hence ultrasonographic surveillance is no longer considered necessary.

Somatostatin analogues are also effective in controlling clinical syndromes associated with unresectable pancreatic NETs, including vasoactive intestinal peptide-producing tumours (VIPomas), glucagonomas and occasionally insulinomas, although 50% of the latter demonstrate a paradoxical fall in blood glucose levels because of suppression of counter-regulatory hormones such as glucagon. However, proton pump inhibitors form the mainstay of medical therapy in gastrinomas, with no evidence for added benefit from somatostatin analogue therapy.

Interferon-α

Interferon-α, in a dose of 3–5 MU three to five times weekly, is employed in the treatment of NETs, either alone or more commonly in combination with somatostatin analogue therapy. However, its use is not widespread at present, in part related to conflicting data as to its efficacy in addition to difficulties with tolerability and high cost. Nevertheless, biochemical and symptomatic response may be seen in 40–70% of patients, and it may be particularly effective in combination with somatostatin analogues and in tumours that are slowly proliferative.

Chemotherapy

The precise role of chemotherapy and the most effective chemotherapeutic regimen in NETs remain uncertain and are areas of active research currently. Suffice to say that at present it is clear that well-differentiated, slowly proliferating gut NETs do not benefit from chemotherapy, whereas poorly differentiated, rapidly growing lesions may exhibit up to 70% response rate with cisplatin and etoposide combinations. Bronchial NETs are also often treated with combinations of platinum and etoposide, while pancreatic NETs may show response rates of 40–70% using combinations of 5-fluorouracil, streptozotocin, dacarbazine and doxorubicin (Adriamycin).

Radionuclide therapy

Because NETs are relatively radioresistant, there is a limited role for conventional external beam radiotherapy in their treatment other than for pain relief in bony metastases. However, by targeting radiodelivery directly to the tumour sites, higher doses of radiation can be administered than with beam radiation, multiple sites can be treated simultaneously and non-target damage can be minimized. Targeted radionuclide therapy can be used for symptomatic patients with unresectable or metastatic disease when abnormally increased uptake of the corresponding imaging compound is evident, provided that patients are not pregnant, breast feeding or have significant myelosuppression or renal failure. Gamma-emitting radionuclides are replaced by beta emitters (such as iodine-131 MIBG, yttrium-90 octreotide or yttrium-90 lanreotide). Therapy is available only at a limited number of centres currently and trials are still ongoing, although early results highlight the considerable promise of this technique, with significant benefits in terms of symptom control, biochemical response and tumour stabilization.

Embolization and radiofrequency ablation

Embolization of the hepatic artery may be indicated for patients with multiple and hormonally active liver metastases that are not amenable to surgical resection. The aim of therapy is to control symptoms and reduce tumour size. The methods used vary considerably, but the technique can utilize various combinations of embolizing particles, chemotherapeutic agents and radionuclides, and in-house guidelines should be developed at each centre. Symptomatic response occurs in 40–80% of patients, but potential therapeutic benefit should be balanced against a recognized mortality of 4–7% and possible side-effects including postembolization syndrome (fever, abdominal pain and nausea), carcinoid crisis (the risk of which should be minimized by octreotide infusion, judicious use of fluids, antibiotics and allopurinol) and hepatic abscess formation (5%). Only one lobe is embolized per session, and patients should be carefully selected to ensure patency of the portal vein and adequate liver function.

Radiofrequency ablation, which may be performed laparoscopically or percutaneously, is an emerging technique that has been used successfully in managing colorectal liver metastases. There is considerably less experience with its use in neuroendocrine liver metastases, although symptomatic improvement can occur when at least 90% of the visible tumour is ablated.

INHERITED ENDOCRINE CANCER SYNDROMES

Multiple endocrine neoplasia

Multiple endocrine neoplasia type 1

Definition and genetics

Multiple endocrine neoplasia type 1 has a wide phenotypic expression (Table 9.4), although three tumour types predominate:

1. parathyroid adenomas
2. enteropancreatic endocrine tumours
3. pituitary adenomas.

The presence of two of these three main tumours in an individual patient establishes a working diagnosis of MEN-1. Familial MEN-1 is defined on the basis of an index MEN-1 case plus at least one relative affected by one of the three main tumours (see Box 9.1). It has an estimated prevalence of one in 10 000 and is inherited as an autosomal dominant trait with high penetrance. The MEN-1 gene is located on chromosome 11q13 and was identified by positional cloning in 1997. Tumours from patients with MEN-1 possess germline mutations in the MEN-1 gene plus a second somatic 'hit' involving 11q13, in keeping with Knudson's two-hit model of tumorigenesis and the postulated role of MEN-1 as a tumour suppressor gene. The cloning of the MEN-1 gene has

221

'cure' to only a small percentage of patients. However, where surgery is considered, selective angiography with secretagogue injection may be particularly useful in biochemical localization in patients with MEN-1, as different tumours may coexist.

Insulinomas are the second commonest of the functional enteropancreatic tumours in MEN-1 and should be investigated and treated as for sporadic tumours, although selective angiography may again prove particularly helpful in confirming the source of insulin excess in multiple islet disease.

The management of asymptomatic non-functioning enteropancreatic tumours in MEN-1 is controversial, although many centres now recommend surgery if one tumour is more than 2 cm in size.

Other manifestations

Foregut carcinoids in MEN-1 typically occur in the bronchial tree, thymus and stomach, although they are not generally hormone-secreting. Thymic carcinoids present more frequently in male patients (and can exhibit markedly aggressive behaviour), whereas bronchial carcinoids are typically seen in female patients. Consensus views suggest that both tumours should be screened for by triennial CT scans. Type 2 gastric carcinoids occur in MEN-1 patients with Zollinger–Ellison syndrome. They arise from enterochromaffin-like cells and are usually small and multiple. Little is known about their malignant potential, but most centres do not presently undertake endoscopic surveillance and therapy principally involves control of hypergastrinaemia using proton pump inhibitors.

Adrenal cortical tumours are often identified on abdominal imaging in MEN-1, but these are rarely functional and usually follow a benign course. There is little consensus on the management of these tumours at present. Cutaneous lesions, including lipomas and facial angiofibromas, are present in a high proportion of patients.

Screening in MEN-1 carriers

Although screening has not yet been shown to improve outcome in MEN-1 (in contrast to MEN-2), definite or likely carriers of MEN-1 mutations are likely to benefit from early identification of tumour expression. Tests should begin in a stepwise fashion in childhood, and comprise annual biochemistry with less frequent imaging. A consensus view on the modality and frequency of biochemical and radiological tests is summarized in Table 9.5, although the precise schedule used in individual centres will be partly dependent on local availability and cost.

Multiple endocrine neoplasia type 2

Definition and genetics

Multiple endocrine neoplasia type 2 is an autosomal dominant syndrome characterized by MTC, phaeochromocytoma and parathyroid tumours. The condition may be further divided along phenotypic lines into MEN-2a (the commonest presentation, accounting for 75% of cases) and several rare variants including familial MTC, MEN-2a with cutaneous lichen amyloidosis, MEN-2a with Hirschsprung's disease and MEN-2b (Table 9.6). MEN-2 occurs because of germline mutations in the RET gene on chromosome 10; DNA testing is widely available and sequencing can usually be restricted to just six of the 21 exons (exons 10, 11 and 13–16), as only a limited range of mutations have been described (Table 9.7). In contrast to MEN-1, MEN-2 shows a strong genotype–phenotype correlation (Table 9.7). This has important practical implications, particularly in relation to the timing of prophylactic thyroidectomy (see below). Treatment may therefore be individualized according to the particular RET codon mutation.

Table 9.6: Classification of multiple endocrine neoplasia type 2

MEN-2 subtype	Phenotype
MEN-2a	MTC (100%) Phaeochromocytoma (50%) Parathyroid tumours (20%)
Familial MTC	MTC only
MEN-2a with cutaneous lichen amyloidosis	MEN-2a Pruritic lesion over upper back
MEN-2a with Hirschsprung's disease	MEN-2a Hirschsprung's disease
MEN-2b	MTC (100%) Phaeochromocytoma (50%) No parathyroid disease Intestinal and mucosal ganglioneuromas Marfanoid body habitus

MEN, multiple endocrine neoplasia; MTC, medullary thyroid carcinoma.

Table 9.7: Genotype–phenotype relationship in multiple endocrine neoplasia type 2[a]

Codon mutation	Syndrome
609 611 618 620 634	MEN-2a/familial MTC
634 768 791 804	MEN-2a/cutaneous lichen amyloidosis Familial MTC
609 618 620	MEN-2a/Hirschsprung's disease
918	MEN-2b

MEN, multiple endocrine neoplasia; MTC, medullary thyroid carcinoma.
[a]Mutations in codon 634 account for 85% of all MEN-2a mutations. Rare mutations have also been described in codons 630, 883, 891 and 922.

Medullary thyroid carcinoma in MEN-2

Medullary thyroid carcinoma is a malignant tumour of the calcitonin-secreting C cells and is preceded by C-cell hyperplasia in MEN-2, a process that may take several years. Premature death from metastatic MTC was common in MEN-2 prior to the introduction of detection strategies centred on calcitonin measurement in the 1970s. These have now been superseded by RET mutational analysis following an improved understanding of MTC behaviour according to genotype and the recognition that stimulated calcitonin testing is less sensitive and specific than previously thought. Furthermore, with the observation that microscopic MTC can develop in very early childhood, management strategies have changed to recommend earlier intervention. Therefore patients with MEN-2 may be classified into three groups of risk according to RET genotype.

- Level 3 (highest risk) patients (codons 883, 918 and 922 or MEN-2b) should undergo total thyroidectomy and central lymph node dissection within the first 6 months of life or at the time of presentation.
- Level 2 (high risk) patients (codons 611, 618, 620, 634 and 891) should undergo surgery before age 5 years.
- Level 1 (intermediate risk) patients (codons 609, 768, 790, 791 and 804) have the least high risk and may generally undergo total thyroidectomy at a later age, although opinion differs as to whether this should be by age 5 years as in level 2 patients, by age 10 years, or based on results of periodic pentagastrin-stimulated calcitonin testing.

Following successful surgery, all patients should undergo annual calcitonin testing (basal or stimulated).

Phaeochromocytoma

Approximately 50% of MEN-2 carriers will develop a phaeochromocytoma, and tumours have been identified in patients as young as 5 years. Bilateral disease is not uncommon, although malignancy seems to be rare. Screening, which should begin at the age of 5 years, should comprise annual measurement of 24-h urinary catecholamines or metadrenaline (metepinephrine; phaeochromocytomas in MEN-2 often preferentially secrete adrenaline [epinephrine] and its metabolites) followed by imaging (MRI, CT, MIBG) when elevated as in sporadic disease. Laparoscopic adrenalectomy is frequently possible, as many tumours will be detected early (<2 cm) with prospective screening.

Parathyroid tumours

Hyperparathyroidism occurs in 20% of patients with MEN-2 (typically with codon 634 mutations) but usually runs a milder course than in MEN-1. The criteria for establishing the diagnosis and for surgical intervention are as for sporadic disease (see Ch. 4); many surgeons perform a subtotal parathyroidectomy to leave a remnant of parathyroid tissue, as recurrent hyperparathyroidism is rare.

Genetic diseases predisposing to phaeochromocytoma and paraganglioma

Phaeochromocytomas were traditionally thought to have an inherited basis in 10% of patients, but following the discovery of the role of the succinate dehydrogenase (SDH) gene family in familial phaeochromocytoma/paraganglioma, revised estimates put this figure at closer to 25%. Phaeochromocytomas and paragangliomas are now recognized as being associated with MEN-2, VHL, NF-1 and phaeochromocytoma/paraganglioma syndrome from mutations in SDHB, SDHD or rarely SDHC. Phaeochromocytoma may also be a component of MEN-1, but this is extremely uncommon (0.5%).

Von Hippel–Lindau syndrome is an autosomal dominant condition characterized by retinal and central nervous system haemangioblastomas, phaeochromocytomas, renal cell carcinomas and renal/pancreatic cysts. VHL may be classified further according to phenotypic expression into:

- type 1 (families with haemangioblastoma and renal cell carcinomas but not phaeochromocytoma)
- type 2a (haemangioblastoma, phaeochromocytoma, low-risk renal cell carcinomas)
- type 2b (haemangioblastoma, phaeochromocytoma, high-risk renal cell carcinomas)
- type 2c (phaeochromocytoma alone).

The overall frequency of phaeochromocytoma in VHL is 20% (bilateral disease in 40%), but patients harbouring missense mutations may be particularly prone to early-onset and extra-adrenal disease. Tumours may preferentially secrete noradrenaline (norepinephrine) and normetadrenaline (normetepinephrine) because of absent expression of phenylethanolamine-N-methyltransferase, which catalyses the conversion of noradrenaline to adrenaline, and this may serve as a clue to the diagnosis. Phaeochromocytoma patients identified as having VHL should be entered into a surveillance programme consisting of annual urinalysis, fundoscopy and 24-h urinary catecholamines, and triennial brain and abdominal MRI.

Mutations in three of the four mitochondrial complex 2 subunit genes (SDH subunits B, C and D but not SDH subunit A) have recently been described in association with hereditary phaeochromocytoma/paraganglioma syndromes. Of these, SDHB and SDHD are the most relevant to endocrinologists, as SDHC mutations have not yet been described as predisposing to phaeochromocytoma (head and neck paraganglioma described in a few families only). Mutations of both SDHB and SDHD are associated with head and neck paragangliomas and phaeochromocytoma, with comparatively high rates of extra-adrenal versus adrenal disease. However, SDHB mutations seem to predispose to aggressive tumours and a greater risk of malignancy. There are also differences evident in the mode of inheritance of the two genes: SDHB is an autosomal dominant disease, whereas SDHD shows evidence of maternal imprinting, i.e. phaeochromocytoma or paraganglioma develops only when the gene is paternally transmitted. Renal cell carcinoma has also been reported in SDHB-associated disease, but reports of papillary thyroid carcinoma in two patients (one with SDHB, one with SDHD) must be viewed with caution at present. Identification of a mutation in an affected individual should lead to regular screening for associated tumours and to consideration of genetic testing in first-degree relatives. Although there is currently little consensus on a recommended surveillance programme for mutation carriers, patients should be reviewed annually for measurement of blood pressure and 24-h urinary fractionated metanephrines or free catecholamines, and biennially for MRI of the neck, thorax, abdomen and pelvis. Screening may need to begin from as early as age 5–10 years for SDHB mutation carriers.

Phaeochromocytomas occur in less than 5% of patients with NF-1, but analysis for germline mutations in the NF-1 gene in patients with apparently sporadic phaeochromocytoma is not justified (the coding region is very large) unless a careful clinical examination raises suspicion (café au lait patches, neurofibromas, axillary freckling).

Most patients with phaeochromocytoma present with apparently sporadic disease and no obvious disease manifestations of VHL, MEN-2, NF-1 or phaeochromocytoma/paraganglioma syndrome. However, a number of studies have recently shown that germline mutations in VHL, RET, SDHB or SDHD are present in 15–25% of such cases. Genetic testing for these conditions may therefore need to be considered in all phaeochromocytomas, but in practice this is restricted to young patients (<50 years) or those presenting with malignant, bilateral or extra-adrenal disease.

Familial isolated hyperparathyroidism and the hyperparathyroidism–jaw tumour syndrome

Most patients with primary hyperparathyroidism have sporadic disease, although rarely the condition forms part of a wider hereditary endocrine tumour syndrome. A number of syndromes have been described in this context, including MEN-1 and MEN-2, familial hypocalciuric hypercalcaemia (see Ch. 4), hyperparathyroidism–jaw tumour syndrome and familial isolated hyperparathyroidism (FIHP). Hyperparathyroidism–jaw tumour syndrome is an autosomal dominant condition associated with germline mutations in the HRPT-2 gene (encoding a protein termed *parafibromin*). The syndrome comprises parathyroid adenoma (characteristically aggressive with cystic appearances on histology) or carcinoma (in 15%), and ossifying fibromas of the mandible or maxilla (in 30% of patients). Renal cysts, Wilms tumour and uterine abnormalities may also be apparent in a proportion of affected families. When parathyroid tumours are the sole manifestation in an affected family, then this is termed *FIHP*, although it is important to recognize that apparent FIHP may represent incomplete expression of another syndrome (e.g. MEN-1 mutations described in up to 18%). FIHP is therefore a diagnosis of exclusion, and affected families may need to undergo genetic testing for mutations in MEN-1 or HRPT-2 depending on the clinical presentation. HRPT-2 mutational testing should particularly be considered in families with parathyroid carcinoma or adenoma with cystic change.

Carney complex

Carney complex is an autosomal dominant syndrome combining spotty skin pigmentation (typically a centrofacial distribution involving the lips and conjunctiva), cardiac myxomas, peripheral nerve lesions (psammomatous melanotic schwannoma) and a number of endocrine disorders. Cushing's syndrome appears to be the commonest endocrine manifestation, affecting up to a third of patients. Uniquely, this occurs because of primary pigmented nodular adrenal disease, a disorder characterized by bilateral, multiple, small, pigmented adrenal nodules that are visible on CT or MRI. Patients are often diagnosed with Cushing's syndrome in adolescence, although the presentation may be atypical, with short stature, osteoporosis and muscle wasting occasionally dominating rather than obesity. The 24-hour urinary cortisol production may also be normal or only mildly elevated, but the diurnal rhythm of serum cortisol is lost. Adrenocorticotrophic hormone levels are suppressed, and the treatment is bilateral adrenalectomy.

Growth hormone-secreting tumours giving rise to acromegaly occur in 10% of patients, and testicular tumours (classically a large cell calcifying Sertoli cell tumour) affect a third of male patients. Ovarian tumours and thyroid follicular neoplasms (benign and malignant) are also components of the complex.

Cowden's syndrome

Cowden's syndrome is an autosomal dominant condition, characterized by multiple hamartomas, which arises from germline mutations in the phosphatase and tensin homologue deleted on chromosome 10 (PTEN) gene. Although rare (estimated gene frequency of one per million), endocrinologists may recognize the condition in patients presenting with multinodular goitre, thyroid carcinoma (particularly follicular carcinoma, rarely papillary but never medullary) or thyroid adenoma. Carcinoma of the breast represents the most serious component tumour (20–50% lifetime risk), but benign breast lesions (fibrocystic disease) occur more commonly. Mucocutaneous lesions, comprising trichilemmomas, verucoid papules and acral keratoses, are characteristic of the syndrome and are present in 90–100% of subjects. Endocrinologists should be particularly suspicious of the condition when young patients present with multifocal thyroid disease, in which case a careful history and physical examination should be undertaken.

McCune–Albright syndrome

McCune–Albright syndrome is a syndrome that occurs because of somatic mutation within the GNAS-1 gene, resulting in activation of G-protein α chains. It is characterized by the triad of polyostotic fibrous dysplasia, café au lait pigmentation and multiple endocrinopathies. The bony lesions develop in childhood and may cause deformity, fractures or nerve entrapment. The café au lait patches have an irregular border (said to resemble the coast of Maine, in contrast to NF-1, in which they resemble the coast of California) and are ipsilateral to the fibrous dysplasia. Precocious puberty is the commonest endocrine manifestation (especially in girls), but fertility is usually retained. Growth hormone excess is also relatively common (30%) and may cause gigantism or acromegaly. Hyperprolactinaemia frequently coexists (over 50%), but only 65% of patients have radiographic evidence of a pituitary adenoma. Treatment involves surgery, dopamine agonists or somatostatin analogues. Thyroid nodules are nearly always present on ultrasonography but are rarely palpable; a third of patients will develop autonomous hyperfunction, causing hyperthyroidism. Treatment may involve antithyroid drugs, radioiodine therapy or surgery. Cushing's syndrome from adrenal gland hyperplasia or solitary adenoma occurs less commonly (usually presenting at a young age). Hypophosphataemic rickets, which occurs because of hyperphosphaturia, is also rare.

Further reading

Benn DE, Robinson BG 2006 Genetic basis of phaeochromocytoma and paraganglioma. Best Pract Res Clin Endocrinol Metab 20: 435–450

Brandi ML, Gagel RF, Angeli A et al. 2001 Guidelines for diagnosis and therapy of MEN type 1 and type 2. J Clin Endocrinol Metab 86: 5658–5671

Plockinger U, Rindi G, Arnold R et al. for the European Neuroendocrine Tumour Society 2004 Guidelines for the diagnosis and treatment of neuroendocrine gastrointestinal tumours. A consensus statement on behalf of the European Neuroendocrine Tumour Society (ENETS). Neuroendocrinology 80: 394–424

Ramage JK, Davies AHG, Ardill J et al. for the UKNETwork for Neuroendocrine Tumours 2005 Guidelines for the management of gastroenteropancreatic neuroendocrine (including carcinoid) tumours. Gut 54: 1–16

SELF-ASSESSMENT

Patient 1

A 40-year-old gentleman, with no significant previous medical history, presents with a 1-year history of 10-kg weight loss and a rash involving the perineum, extremities (Fig. 9.6a) and sites of minor trauma. The lesions show erosive erythema, are occasionally bullous, and heal with crusting and pigmentation. He has a glossy tongue (Fig. 9.6b), but examination is otherwise unremarkable.

Figure 9.6
Patient 1: **(a)** rash, **(b)** glossy tongue, **(c)** abdominal computerized tomography scan.

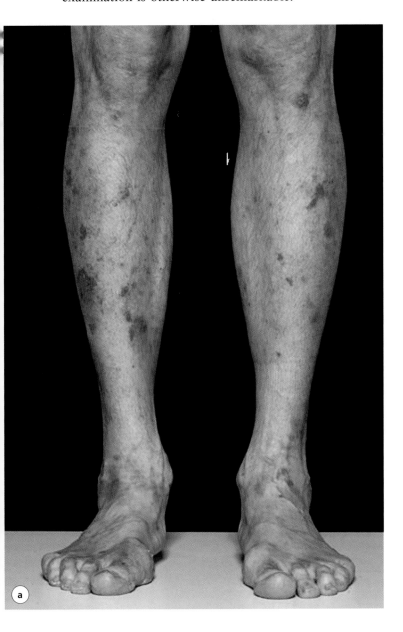

Figure 9.6—cont'd

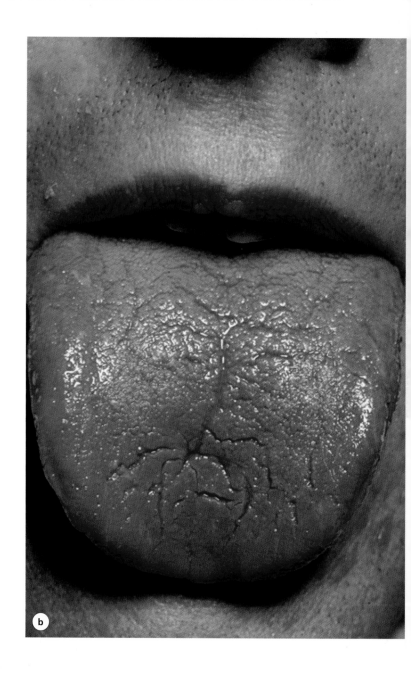

Questions
1. What is the differential diagnosis of the rash?
2. What investigations would you arrange?

Answers
1. The rash has all the hallmarks of a deficiency dermatosis. The differential
   dermatological diagnosis would include necrolytic migratory erythema, zinc deficiency
   and necrolytic acral erythema. Pellagra can have similar histological appearances to

Figure 9.6—cont'd

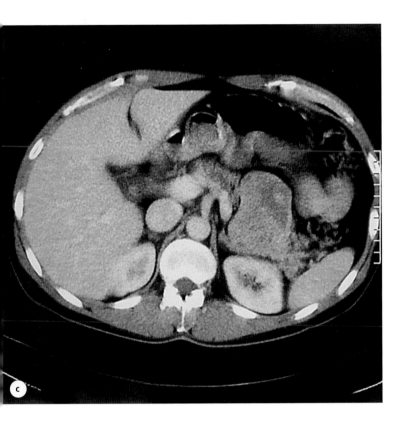

these conditions, but the rash is present in sun-exposed areas, symmetrical, sharply demarcated and particularly prominent over the hands, arms and face. Necrolytic acral erythema is strongly associated with hepatitis C.

2. A skin biopsy showed vacuolated keratinocytes in the upper epidermis, leading to confluent necrosis. He had a mild normocytic anaemia, but renal function, liver function, electrolyte status and random glucose were all normal. An abdominal CT scan was performed (Fig. 9.6c).

Questions
3. What does the CT scan show?
4. What other investigations would you organize?
5. What treatment modalities are available for this condition?

Answers
3. The CT scan shows a large (7 cm) mass in the pancreatic tail. There was no evidence of lymph node or distant metastases.
4. An octreotide scan confirmed a solitary 'hotspot' corresponding to the mass visible on CT. Further biochemistry demonstrated hypoaminoacidaemia, an elevated serum CgA and a fasting glucagon of 375 pmol/L (normal <50 pmol/L), confirming the diagnosis of glucagonoma.

233

Figure 9.7
Patient 2: **(a)** chest x-ray, **(b)** metaiodobenzylguanidine scan.

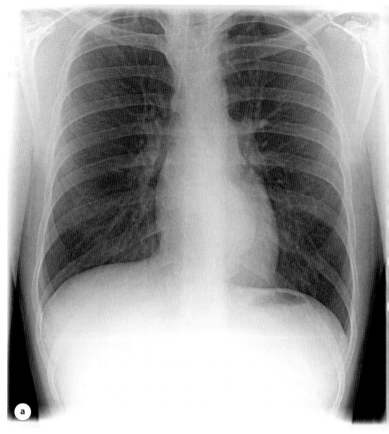

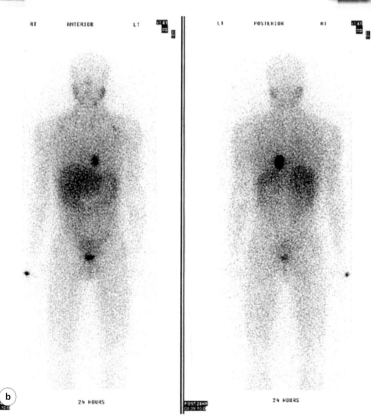

234

5. The patient underwent a distal pancreatectomy and splenectomy. The rash disappeared almost immediately, the glucagon concentration returned to normal, and he regained the weight that he had lost. He remains well, with normal glucagon levels, at 3 years' follow-up. Glucagonoma frequently presents with metastases; the tumour is resistant to chemotherapy, and surgical resection may not be possible in such circumstances. Nevertheless, survival can be prolonged because the tumour is usually slow-growing. Long-acting somatostatin analogues can provide good palliation, with or without interferon-α therapy. In some cases, zinc, amino acid and fatty acid supplementation may also be beneficial.

Patient 2

A 16-year-old boy presents with an episode of vomiting and prolonged pallor following a period of exercise. He is found to be hypertensive (150/90 mmHg), and a chest x-ray is performed (Fig. 9.7a).

Question
1. What does the chest x-ray show?

Answer
1. There is a retrocardiac shadow present.

On detailed review, the patient gives a history of intermittent attacks of nausea, giddiness, perspiration and pallor occurring particularly after exercise. There is no relevant family history, and he denies significant headache or palpitations.

Questions
2. What other investigations would you arrange?
3. How should he be treated?

Answers
2. A CT scan of the neck, thorax and abdomen showed a solitary mass in the thorax corresponding to the lesion evident on his chest x-ray; a 24-h urine collection revealed a markedly raised noradrenaline (norepinephrine) level (10 540 nmol; normal 100–820 nmol), confirming the diagnosis of a paraganglioma. An iodine-123 MIBG scan demonstrated a solitary area of increased uptake in the thoracic lesion only (Fig. 9.7b).
3. The patient was begun on consecutive alpha (phenoxybenzamine) and beta (propranolol) blockade for a few weeks prior to surgery. Surgical resection was complete, his hypertension resolved and repeat urine catecholamines have been persistently normal. He underwent genetic testing for germline mutations in RET, VHL, SDHB and SDHD. This demonstrated a frameshift mutation in exon 4 of the SDHB gene. Family screening is under way, while his urinalysis and baseline MRI scan of the neck, thorax, abdomen and pelvis were normal. This should be repeated biennially.

Endocrine emergencies

10

A. Rees

THYROTOXIC CRISIS

This is a rare and severe form of hyperthyroidism that requires early diagnosis and treatment in view of its high mortality (up to 50% in some series). Its incidence seems to be declining, probably because of a combination of factors including earlier recognition and treatment and better preparation of patients undergoing surgery or ablative radioiodine therapy for hyperthyroidism. A high index of suspicion should be maintained, as clinical signs and symptoms are often non-specific and may be masked in the elderly; they may include:

- pyrexia
- confusion
- agitation
- tachycardia
- diarrhoea and vomiting
- jaundice.

These symptoms may be present in addition to signs of thyrotoxicosis (goitre, Graves' ophthalmopathy) or multisystem decompensation (cardiac failure, respiratory distress, dehydration) (Box 10.1). A careful history is also mandatory to identify possible precipitants, such as amiodarone treatment, recent antithyroid drug withdrawal, iodine-131 therapy, administration of iodinated contrast agents, sepsis, surgery (thyroidal or non-thyroidal) or recent pregnancy.

Investigations may reveal a leucocytosis, minor hypercalcaemia and a raised alkaline phosphatase, in addition to raised thyroid hormones and suppressed thyroid-stimulating hormone (TSH), although the rise in circulating free triiodothyronine (T_3) and free thyroxine (T_4) in thyroid storm is often of the same order of magnitude as in uncomplicated thyrotoxicosis and cannot be used to distinguish between the two states. Also, very sick patients may demonstrate a 'euthyroid sick' syndrome in which thyroid hormone levels may be lower than anticipated.

Because of the high morbidity and mortality associated with this condition, treatment should not be delayed pending the results of thyroid function tests. Treatment comprises general supportive measures in addition to specific therapy targeted to the thyroid gland.

Patients should be treated in a critical care environment with appropriate monitoring of temperature, fluid balance, cardiac, respiratory and neurological status.

Supportive measures

Dehydration should be treated vigorously with fluid resuscitation, used judiciously in elderly patients or those with signs of cardiac compromise. Fluid replacement will usually correct any associated hypercalcaemia that may be present. Pyrexia should be treated with paracetamol (acetaminophen) and external cooling. Chlorpromazine, which is useful to treat agitation, may have the added benefit of reducing fever because of its central inhibitory thermoregulatory properties. Congestive cardiac failure and tachyarrhythmias should be treated in the usual manner, although greater than normal doses of digoxin may be required and hypokalaemia must be corrected first. Patients with thyrotoxicosis and atrial arrhythmias are at particular risk of thrombotic complications and should receive anticoagulation with heparin and warfarin in the absence of any contraindications. In fact, prophylactic anticoagulation is probably indicated even in the absence of dysrhythmias, as thrombotic risk (notably cerebral venous sinus thrombosis) may be increased in thyrotoxicosis alone. Hypotension may require inotropic support on a temporary basis, and corticosteroids are frequently given (usually in the form of intravenous hydrocortisone 100 mg 8-hourly), not only on the basis of possible relative adrenal insufficiency but also for their ability to block the conversion of T_4 to T_3. A search for possible precipitants should include an infection screen (cultures of urine, blood and sputum) and merits empirical therapy with broad-spectrum antibiotics in most cases.

Antithyroid therapy

Thionamides are given, usually in high doses and by mouth or nasogastric tube (rectal preparations of both carbimazole and propylthiouracil are also available), to inhibit the synthesis of new thyroid hormones completely. Propylthiouracil is generally preferred, as it has the added benefit of blocking the conversion of T_4 to T_3 in the periphery. Typical initial doses are 1200–1500 mg of propylthiouracil daily (given in divided doses 4–6 hourly) or 120 mg of carbimazole daily (in divided doses 4–6 hourly). The continued release of preformed thyroid hormone must also be addressed, typically by giving Lugol's solution (eight drops every 6 h) or a solution of potassium iodide (60 mg every 6 h), although lithium carbonate (given initially as 300 mg every 6 h, with subsequent dose adjustment to maintain serum lithium levels at about 1 mmol/L) can also be used for this purpose in those with a history of allergy to iodine. It is imperative that iodine is administered after thionamide therapy has been commenced (at least 4 h later), as iodine use without prior thionamide treatment will enrich thyroid hormone stores, potentially exacerbating the thyrotoxicosis. The combination of iodine with thionamide usually restores circulating thyroid hormone concentrations to normal within 4–5 days. It is worth noting that amiodarone-induced thyroid crisis demands a different approach, and this is discussed in Chapter 3.

The peripheral manifestations of thyroid hormone excess are best treated with β-adrenergic blockade, usually in the form of propranolol given in high doses orally (60–120 mg every 6 h) or intravenously (2–5 mg/h). The cardiac rhythm should be monitored closely, and beta blockers may need to be used cautiously in patients with significant left ventricular impairment. Beta blockers will also help control agitation, tremor, fever and diarrhoea when present. In those with a history of bronchospasm, some success has been reported with the very short-acting cardioselective beta blocker esmolol, or alternatively a rate-limiting calcium channel blocker such as diltiazem could be used. In patients refractory to these above measures, enhanced disposal of excess circulating thyroid hormone can be achieved through peritoneal dialysis or plasmapheresis. Figure 10.1 summarizes the key components of a management strategy for thyroid storm.

MYXOEDEMA COMA

Myxoedema coma is a rare, extreme manifestation of the hypothyroid state and typically affects elderly women with long-standing but frequently unrecognized or untreated hypothyroidism. The mortality rate is notably high (up to 60%) despite early diagnosis and treatment, and its management involves a multisystem approach in an intensive care setting. The history in such patients should explore potential precipitants such as infection, drugs (sedatives, antidepressants, opiates, lithium, amiodarone), and cerebrovascular or cardiac disease, in addition to direct clues to a thyroid aetiology such as previous thyroidectomy, ablative radioiodine therapy or discontinuation of T_4 replacement (Box 10.2). Physical examination may reveal bradycardia, dry skin, macroglossia, a goitre, hyporeflexia, hypoventilation and evidence of cardiac failure, in

Administer i.v. fluids[a]

- Obtain blood for free T_3, free T_4 and TSH measurements
- Check blood cultures, electrolyte status and renal function
- Correct hypokalaemia when present

- Begin paracetamol (acetaminophen) for fever; externally cool
- Consider chlorpromazine for agitation (50mg p.o./i.m.)

If vomiting, pass nasogastric tube

- Control tachycardia with propranolol[b] (60-120mg every 6h p.o or i.v. infusion at 2-5mg/h)
- Consider high-dose digoxin
- Anticoagulate if atrial arrhythmia

Give i.v. hydrocortisone (100mg every 6-8h)

- Begin propylthiouracil (e.g. 300mg every 6h p.o. or via nasogastric tube)
- Add Lugol's solution *after* 4h (eight drops every 6h)

Treat infection with broad-spectrum antibiotics

Figure 10.1
Management of thyrotoxic crisis. All patients should be treated in a critical care environment with close monitoring of fluid balance, temperature, cardiac, respiratory and neurological status. [a]Fluids should be used cautiously in those with significant cardiac impairment. [b]In the absence of any contraindications. Esmolol or rate-limiting calcium channel blockers may be suitable alternatives. T_3, triiodothyronine; T_4, thyroxine; TSH, thyroid-stimulating hormone.

Box 10.2: Presenting symptoms, signs and identifiable precipitants in myxoedema coma

Symptoms and signs

- Altered mental state: confusion, psychosis, coma
- Hypothermia (often profound)
- Respiratory depression, airway obstruction
- Cardiomegaly, bradycardia, hypotension, pleural effusion, ascites
- Abdominal pain, distension, constipation
- Hyporeflexia
- Dry skin, macroglossia, goitre, neck scar

Precipitants

- Infection
- Drugs (antidepressants, anaesthetics, sedatives, opiates, lithium, amiodarone)
- Cardiac or cerebrovascular disease
- Hypothermia
- Trauma
- Discontinuation of thyroxine replacement therapy

---

addition to the cardinal signs of hypothermia, which is often profound, and coma (Box 10.2).

Laboratory findings may include hyponatraemia, hypoglycaemia, anaemia, hypercholesterolaemia, hypoxia and/or hypercapnia and an elevated creatine kinase level, while an electrocardiogram (ECG) may demonstrate low-voltage complexes, bradycardia, varying degrees of heart block, T-wave inversion and prolongation of the QT interval. Thyroid function tests, which may suggest the presence of a pituitary or hypothalamic basis for the hypothyroidism in up to 10% of cases, should be requested urgently, although treatment should not be delayed while awaiting the results.

Treatment centres on intensive supportive measures for the multiple metabolic derangements, coupled with replenishment of thyroid hormone stores. Monitoring of therapy should include frequent assessments of rectal temperature, blood pressure, oxygen saturation, urine output, central venous pressure, arterial blood gas and electrolyte status.

Supportive measures

The most important measure in the immediate setting is to ensure maintenance of an adequate airway to avoid hypoxia. Much of the excess mortality in myxoedema coma relates to respiratory failure, characterized by hypoventilation, carbon dioxide retention and respiratory acidosis. Intubation and mechanical ventilation may need to be considered, especially with worsening hypoxia or hypercapnia, and regular monitoring of arterial blood gases is essential. Warm, humidified oxygen should be given to all patients.

Hypothermia should be corrected by passive external rewarming, although this should not be overly rapid as peripheral vasodilation could ensue, leading to worsening hypotension and shock. Hypotension may need supportive therapy until thyroid hormone supplementation begins to take effect. This should take the form of fluids (5 or 10% dextrose if hypoglycaemia is a concern, or 0.9% saline if hyponatraemia is apparent) used judiciously, as the majority of patients with myxoedema coma are in an age group in which cardiac compromise is frequent. A decision to use inotropes in this setting should involve an assessment of the risk of inotrope-induced ischaemia on the one hand and the adverse outcome of persistent hypotension on the other.

Hyponatraemia, caused by impaired water excretion, can contribute to the comatose state when severe and may require initial therapy with hypertonic saline in this instance, followed by intravenous furosemide to promote a water diuresis. However, in general terms fluid restriction alone is sufficient to correct modest hyponatraemia.

Coexisting adrenal insufficiency may be present in up to 10% of patients (either primary adrenal failure from an autoimmune cause or secondary to pituitary disease) and may be suggested by the characteristic laboratory findings of hyponatraemia, hypoglycaemia, raised urea and hyperkalaemia. For this reason, hydrocortisone should be administered to all patients (initially 100 mg intravenously every 8 h), especially as T_4 replacement can precipitate a crisis in unrecognized adrenal failure. All patients should also receive broad-spectrum antibiotics once appropriate cultures have been obtained.

Thyroid hormone replacement

There is much controversy surrounding the type and mode of thyroid hormone substitution in myxoedema coma, with little evidence to support one regimen over another. Any theoretical benefits surrounding the more rapid physiological effects of T_3 versus T_4 replacement are offset against a greater risk of complications (myocardial

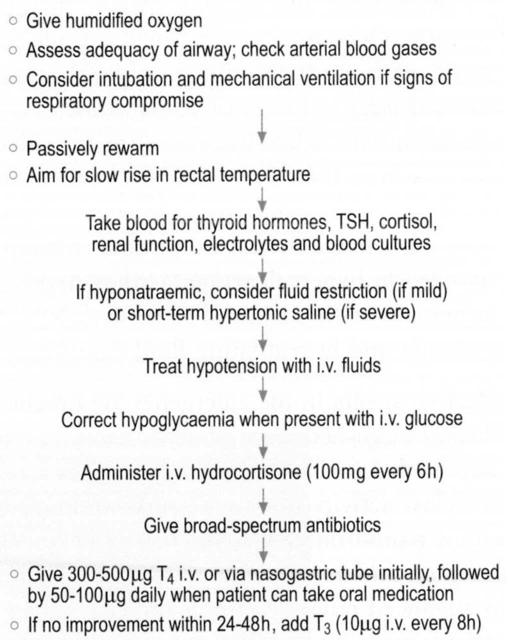

○ Give humidified oxygen

○ Assess adequacy of airway; check arterial blood gases

○ Consider intubation and mechanical ventilation if signs of respiratory compromise

↓

○ Passively rewarm

○ Aim for slow rise in rectal temperature

↓

Take blood for thyroid hormones, TSH, cortisol, renal function, electrolytes and blood cultures

↓

If hyponatraemic, consider fluid restriction (if mild) or short-term hypertonic saline (if severe)

↓

Treat hypotension with i.v. fluids

↓

Correct hypoglycaemia when present with i.v. glucose

↓

Administer i.v. hydrocortisone (100mg every 6h)

↓

Give broad-spectrum antibiotics

↓

○ Give 300-500µg T_4 i.v. or via nasogastric tube initially, followed by 50-100µg daily when patient can take oral medication

○ If no improvement within 24-48h, add T_3 (10µg i.v. every 8h)

Figure 10.2
Management of myxoedema coma. All patients should be treated in a critical care setting with monitoring of the cardiac rhythm, core temperature, fluid balance, cardiac, neurological and respiratory status. T_3, triiodothyronine; T_4, thyroxine; TSH, thyroid-stimulating hormone.

infarction, tachyarrhythmias) with the former. In practice, a compromise is achieved by using T_4 initially, with the subsequent addition of T_3 in cases showing no improvement within 24–48 h. Most authors recommend that this should be in high doses, although limited data suggest that elderly patients tolerate such doses less well, and some would advocate a low-dose regimen in these instances.

Thyroxine is given initially either intravenously or via a nasogastric tube (although aspiration is a concern with the nasogastric route and absorption may be variable), followed by oral administration once the comatose state has resolved. An initial dose of 300–500 µg as a single intravenous bolus is followed by 50–100 µg daily as a maintenance dose. Serum T_3 rises progressively with this regimen because of peripheral conversion from T_4, although associated illness may contribute to a reduced T_4 to T_3 conversion rate from sick euthyroid syndrome. Consequently, failure to witness clinical improvement (and a falling TSH) should prompt clinicians to add intravenous T_3 therapy (10 µg 8-hourly) to the patient's treatment until the patient is well enough to take maintenance T_4. In these circumstances, continuous ECG monitoring (with reduction in dose in the event of arrhythmia or ischaemia) is mandatory. Figure 10.2 summarizes the key management principles in myxoedema coma.

HYPERCALCAEMIA

Severe hypercalcaemia is a life-threatening condition necessitating urgent therapy. Consideration must be given at the outset as to the underlying diagnosis (discussed in

calcium gluconate injection (10 mL of a 10% solution containing 2.25 mmol of calcium). This can be repeated according to symptomatic and biochemical response, although persistent hypocalcaemia requires treatment with a calcium gluconate infusion, titrated according to the serum calcium level. It is mandatory to check the serum magnesium concentration in all patients, as hypocalcaemia will not resolve in uncorrected hypomagnesaemia because of reduced parathyroid hormone secretion and increased parathyroid hormone resistance. In patients who are likely to develop persistent hypocalcaemia, vitamin D replacement should also be commenced.

PITUITARY APOPLEXY

Pituitary apoplexy refers to infarction, often haemorrhagic, of the pituitary gland. Cases typically occur in patients with pituitary macroadenomas, although in most instances these have not been previously recognized. Apoplexy generally occurs spontaneously, although precipitating factors are sometimes apparent and include hypertension, pituitary radiotherapy, postpartum (Sheehan's syndrome) or postcardiac surgery, anticoagulant use, dopamine agonist therapy and dynamic pituitary function testing. Headache, typically severe and usually associated with nausea or vomiting, is almost universal, and up to 80% of patients present with visual deficits. Clinical examination may reveal the presence of bitemporal hemianopia, ocular palsies and altered conscious level. Varying degrees of hypopituitarism are observed in up to 75% of patients at presentation and magnetic resonance imaging (MRI) is the imaging modality of choice (Fig. 10.5).

Management should focus on investigation and treatment of hypopituitarism when present, assessment of neuro-ophthalmological status with close follow-up of visual

Figure 10.5
T_1-weighted magnetic resonance imaging scan in a patient presenting with pituitary apoplexy. Note the high signal intensity typical of haemorrhage.

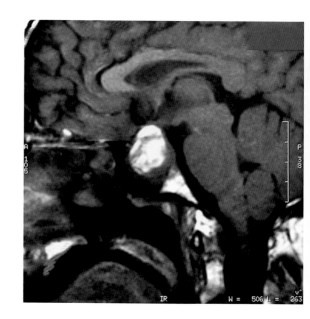

acuity, and possible surgical intervention depending on the severity of presentation and course of the disease. Full assessment of anterior pituitary function, comprising measurement of free T_4, TSH, prolactin, cortisol, gonadotrophins, testosterone/oestradiol and insulin-like growth factor-1, should be performed at baseline. Prolactin levels should be requested urgently in this setting, as apoplexy in the context of macroprolactinomas may respond well to dopamine agonist therapy.

All patients should receive prompt empirical therapy with intravenous hydrocortisone (100 mg 6–8 hourly), and close attention needs to be paid to fluid and electrolyte balance. Pituitary hormone deficiencies should be corrected, but there remains some controversy surrounding the role of decompressive surgery. Recent evidence supports the contention that patients with absent or resolving visual deficit may be treated safely without surgery. However, decompressive surgery should be considered in patients with diminishing level of consciousness or deteriorating visual acuity.

ADRENAL CRISIS

Adrenal crisis falls into a spectrum of presentations ranging from coma and shock on the one hand (hypotension, tachycardia, peripheral vasoconstriction, oliguria) to more subtle signs such as fever, abdominal pain (occasionally due to bilateral adrenal infarction), weakness and confusion. A history of known adrenal insufficiency or recent discontinuation of steroids can be elicited in many but not all patients, and a high index of suspicion for the diagnosis must be maintained.

Therapy for suspected adrenal crisis should begin immediately once the diagnosis is considered, although a request for cortisol and adrenocorticotrophic hormone (ACTH) measurement at presentation (in addition to glucose, urea and electrolytes), prior to hydrocortisone replacement, is useful for later confirmation of the diagnosis. Treatment should not therefore be delayed to accommodate a synacthen test at presentation, although this should be undertaken at a later stage when the patient is stable and the hydrocortisone is temporarily withdrawn. Patients usually have significant reduction in extracellular fluid volume, and immediate treatment should focus on volume repletion with large quantities of intravenous 0.9% saline (several litres in the first 24 h). Hypoglycaemia, which may be evident at presentation or may develop during the course of the illness, should be treated with intravenous glucose.

Hydrocortisone is given intravenously in the first instance (in a dose of 100 mg 6–8 hourly), converting to oral therapy when recovery is in progress, although double the patient's standard replacement dose should be given until full recovery has ensued. Hydrocortisone possesses substantial mineralocorticoid activity in high doses and this, coupled with the large volumes of saline administered, means that oral fludrocortisone (in a dose of 50–100 µg daily) does not need to be commenced until the daily dose of oral hydrocortisone is less than 50 mg. Of course, fludrocortisone does not need to be administered at all in adrenal crisis secondary to pituitary disease, because mineralocorticoid secretion is largely independent of ACTH. A search for precipitants

Figure 10.6
Steroid card and MedicAlert bracelet.

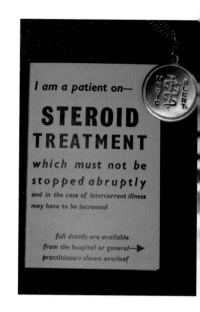

should include a screen for infection, with antibiotic therapy as appropriate, and electrolyte status should be monitored to ensure normalization. Subsequent testing should seek to establish a cause for the adrenal insufficiency, as in the non-acute state (see Ch. 5).

A check should be made prior to discharge from hospital that patients carry a steroid card and/or MedicAlert bracelet (Fig. 10.6), and that they have clear understanding of the need to double or triple hydrocortisone replacement doses at times of intercurrent illness or to seek medical help for intravenous hydrocortisone in the event of protracted diarrhoea or vomiting.

PHAEOCHROMOCYTOMA

Uncontrolled catecholamine release can occasionally occur in patients harbouring a phaeochromocytoma, leading to a pressor crisis. This may occur spontaneously, although a number of precipitants have been identified, including exercise, straining, parturition, abdominal palpation, surgery and drugs (anaesthetics, contrast agents, tricyclic antidepressants, phenothiazines, ACTH, naloxone, morphine, metoclopramide and unopposed beta blockade). In addition to tachycardia and hypertension, which is often marked, patients in crisis may develop:

- chest pain
- myocardial infarction (from coronary vasospasm)
- atrial or ventricular arrhythmias
- overwhelming non-cardiogenic pulmonary oedema.

Neurological complications include hypertensive encephalopathy and cerebrovascular events, and biochemical evidence of glucose intolerance and hypercalcaemia is often apparent. Patients can also develop profound hypotension and acute respiratory distress syndrome, which may be refractory to inotropic support.

In addition to supportive measures, specific treatment involves administration of intravenous boluses of phentolamine (2–5 mg), repeated if necessary to maintain adequate blood pressure control, or alternatively an infusion of sodium nitroprusside. More recently, magnesium sulphate infusions are being recognized as effective in these situations, especially when conventional therapy has failed. Arrhythmias may require therapy with propranolol or esmolol once alpha blockade has been commenced. Once adequate control of hypertension has been established, patients should be commenced on oral phenoxybenzamine, titrating the dose according to postural hypotension and nasal stuffiness, with later addition of a beta blocker such as propranolol to control tachycardia. Patients should then be prepared for surgery.

ACUTE HYPERCORTISOLISM

Cushing's syndrome is frequently associated with neuropsychiatric disturbance, which may take the form of major depression, cognitive impairment, anxiety or psychosis. Occasionally, patients may present in extremis with florid psychosis needing urgent therapy. Patients should be investigated as normal (see Ch. 1) but may need specific medical therapy once the biochemical tests are complete, in order to control the psychosis (and other medical complications) prior to subsequent surgery or while awaiting the effects of radiotherapy.

- Metyrapone, an inhibitor of 11-β-hydroxylase, is usually used first line and is given as a total daily dose of 1–4 g in four divided doses. Doses should be titrated according to control of symptoms and biochemistry (cortisol day curve and urinary free cortisols), being careful to avoid hypoadrenalism (monitor blood glucose and look for postural hypotension). Dexamethasone (0.25 mg t.d.s.) is usually added in a block and replace regimen. Nausea is a common side-effect.
- Ketoconazole (200–400 mg t.d.s.) is an alternative to metyrapone and is often used first line in paediatric Cushing's syndrome. It may take a few weeks to become fully effective, and liver function tests need to be monitored.
- Mifepristone (RU-486) is a glucocorticoid receptor antagonist that is showing considerable promise as an alternative to metyrapone or ketoconazole. Experience is limited, but most reports have used a starting dose of approximately 400 mg/day with gradual increase according to response up to a maximal reported dose of 2 g daily. Adrenal insufficiency is a recognized adverse effect of therapy and demands mifepristone dose reduction plus glucocorticoid administration. However, adrenal insufficiency cannot be confirmed biochemically, because ACTH and cortisol levels are paradoxically increased because of disinhibition of ACTH secretion by pituitary

glucocorticoid receptor blockade. The high circulating cortisol levels may also activate the mineralocorticoid receptor (because of saturation of 11-β-hydroxysteroid dehydrogenase type 2), leading to hypokalaemia and hypertension. Coadministration of spironolactone may therefore be necessary.

- Mitotane is an adrenolytic drug used as adjunctive therapy in adrenal cancer, but its side-effect profile does not make it an attractive option for treatment of acute hypercortisolism.
- Etomidate may be a useful agent if parenteral administration is required.

Further reading

Ayuk J, McGregor EJ, Mitchell RD et al. 2004 Acute management of pituitary apoplexy – surgery or conservative management? Clin Endocrinol 61: 747–752

Burch HB, Wartofsky L 1993 Life-threatening thyrotoxicosis. Thyroid storm. Endocrinol Metab Clin North Am 22: 263–277

Savage MW, Mah PM, Weetman AP et al. 2004 Endocrine emergencies. Postgrad Med J 80: 506–515

SELF-ASSESSMENT

Patient 1

A 33-year-old woman presents to the emergency department with a history of fatigue, syncope, vomiting, productive cough and abdominal pain. Her past medical history is remarkable only for a previous miscarriage at 10 weeks' gestation. Physical examination reveals her to be hypotensive (blood pressure 90/60 mmHg), tachycardic (110/min) and pyrexial (38°C), with bronchial breathing in the right mid-zone and a mildly tender abdomen.

Questions
1. What are the diagnoses and which investigations would you arrange?
2. How should the patient be treated?

Answers
1. The history and examination findings point first to the presence of a community-acquired pneumonia, and initial investigations should seek to confirm this with blood and sputum culture and chest x-ray, and measurement of white cell count, arterial blood gases, renal function and electrolyte status. However, the hypotension and tachycardia and the history of fatigue and syncope should also raise a suspicion of underlying adrenal insufficiency. Electrolyte abnormalities such as hyponatraemia, hyperkalaemia or raised urea and creatinine may provide an additional clue. Blood for cortisol and ACTH (which must be transported quickly to the laboratory for cold centrifugation and freezing) should be taken prior to hydrocortisone administration. Glucose levels should be checked. An underlying cause for the adrenal failure should be considered at presentation, which in this instance, with a history of miscarriage and abdominal pain, may be bilateral haemorrhagic adrenal infarction from primary antiphospholipid antibody syndrome. This diagnosis should be confirmed by measurement of antiphospholipid antibodies and imaging of the adrenal glands by MRI or computerized tomography and, once the acute illness has resolved, subsequent investigation with ACTH (synacthen) stimulation testing.
2. The immediate priorities are fluid resuscitation with large volumes of intravenous 0.9% saline and glucocorticoid replenishment given as 100 mg of intravenous hydrocortisone 6-hourly. When present, hypoglycaemia should be corrected with intravenous glucose, and appropriate antibiotic therapy should be begun for management of the pneumonia. High-flow oxygen should be given, and the patient should be monitored closely in a high-dependency area. The patient should subsequently receive anticoagulation with low molecular weight heparin and warfarin, with tailoring of hydrocortisone dose reduction and introduction of fludrocortisone according to clinical response and subsequent testing. Finally, patient education is of paramount importance prior to hospital discharge.

Patient 2

A 38-year-old morbidly obese lady (140 kg) is admitted to the emergency unit with a history of hallucinations for several months, increasing dyspnoea, productive cough and poor mobility. On arrival, she is extremely unwell with evidence of reduced conscious level, bradycardia, hyporeflexia, macroglossia, hypoventilation (respiratory rate of 10 breaths/min) and hypothermia (core temperature 28°C). The ECG shows a sinus bradycardia with low-voltage QRS complexes in the precordial leads, and laboratory investigations demonstrate hyponatraemia (130 mmol/L) and respiratory acidosis with hypoxia (pH 7.27, p_{CO_2} 8.4 kPa, p_{O_2} 6 kPa).

Questions
1. What is the diagnosis?
2. What possible precipitants should you seek in the history?
3. What are the immediate priorities in her treatment?

Answers
1. The clinical features are all strongly suggestive of myxoedema coma, and urgent treatment should not be delayed while awaiting biochemical confirmation of the diagnosis.
2. A history of recent infection and detailed drug history should be sought, specifically enquiring about sedative, antidepressant, opiate, lithium or amiodarone use. Recent symptoms of respiratory, neurological or cardiac disease should also be recorded, in addition to details of any previous thyroid surgery, prescriptions for thyroid medication (and recent withdrawal) or previous radioiodine therapy.
3. The immediate priority is assessment and stabilization of the patient's airway and respiration. The morbid obesity and macroglossia are likely to cause considerable upper airway obstruction, and there is evidence of significant carbon dioxide narcosis. Intubation and mechanical ventilation are required. With the airway and respiratory system stabilized, priorities can turn to fluid resuscitation, passive external rewarming (aiming for a slow rise in core temperature to avoid circulatory collapse), corticosteroid administration (100 mg hydrocortisone intravenously every 6–8 h initially), broad-spectrum antibiotic therapy, judicious use of inotropic support when necessary, and commencement of high-dose T_4 replacement (300–500 µg of intravenous T_4 in the first 24 h). The ECG should be monitored closely during therapy, alongside assessment of fluid balance, temperature, and neurological and cardiorespiratory function.

Index